THE HEALING
GOUT COOKBOOK

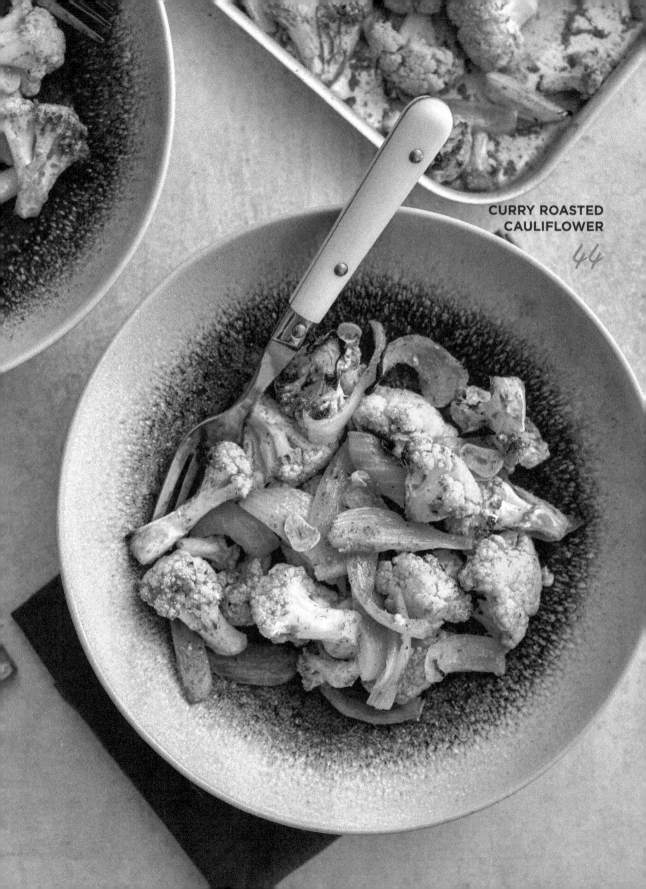

CURRY ROASTED
CAULIFLOWER

44

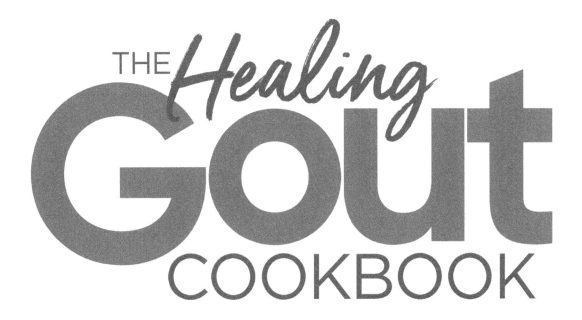

THE Healing GOUT COOKBOOK

ANTI-INFLAMMATORY RECIPES
to Lower Uric Acid Levels
and Reduce Flares

Lisa Cicciarello Andrews, MEd, RD, LD

Photography by Darren Muir

ROCKRIDGE
PRESS

Interior and Cover Designer: Darren Samuel
Art Producer: Karen Williams
Editor: Erum Khan

Photography © Darren Muir, Food styling by Darren Muir, cover and pp. ii, vi, x, 20, 48, 64, 78, 104; © Jennifer Davick, p. 34; © Evi Abeler, p. 92; © Nadine Greeff, p. 116

Author photo courtesy of © Michael Morris

Cover: Fish Tacos with Peach Salsa, p. 73

ISBN: Print 978-1-64611-446-7 | eBook 978-1-64611-447-4

R0

This book is dedicated to my wonderful family—Ryan, Iris, and Maria—who love and support my creative ventures. And to my parents, Frank and Joanne Cicciarello, who taught me to appreciate good food.

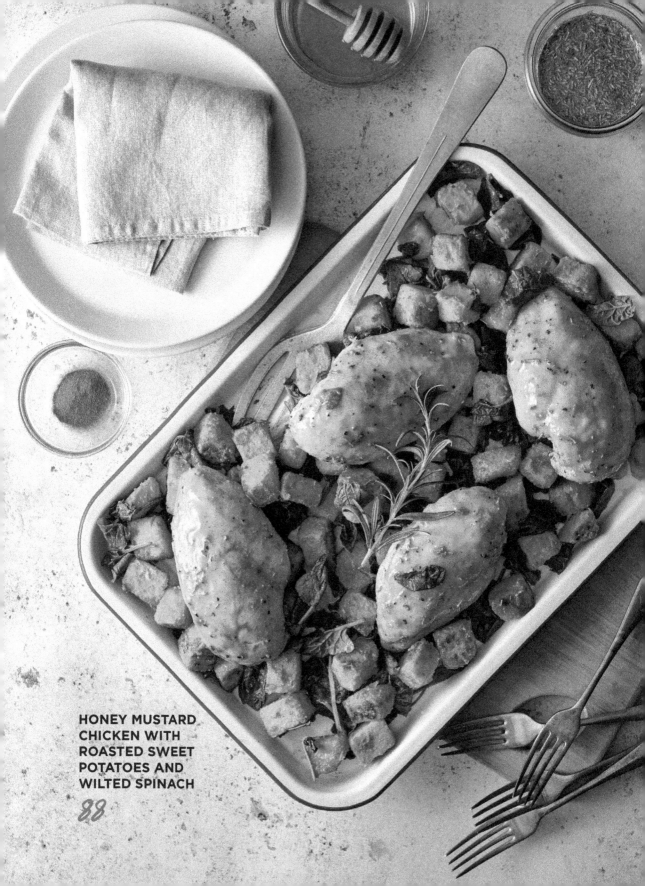

HONEY MUSTARD CHICKEN WITH ROASTED SWEET POTATOES AND WILTED SPINACH

Contents

Introduction

If you've ever experienced a gout flare-up you know how painful it can be. Simple activities like getting dressed, driving, or cooking can be a serious challenge. Gout is just one of hundreds of forms of arthritis and affects up to 4 percent of the population. While gout more commonly impacts older men, women can also suffer gout attacks, particularly after menopause.

During a gout flare-up the last thing you may feel like doing is preparing a meal for yourself or your family. Swollen, painful hands can make it difficult to perform otherwise simple chores like using a can opener or chopping vegetables. Standing on a swollen toe in front of a hot stove, even for a few minutes, can feel like torture to someone with gout. Lack of sleep from a painful joint waking you up in the middle of the night can zap your energy the next day. While you may look perfectly healthy to other people, your pain is *real*.

As a registered dietitian with 30 years in clinical practice, I've witnessed firsthand how difficult living with gout can be. From the frustration of not being able to feed oneself or open a carton of milk to difficulties with getting dressed, gout can really put a damper on someone's life. Gout attacks can come out of nowhere and last a few days—or more than a week. On a personal level, I have lived with rheumatoid arthritis for most of my adult life and understand how debilitating chronic pain can impact quality of life.

But there's good news. You *can* control your gout and experience relief from this painful arthritic condition. Research shows that a healthy, low-purine diet may aid in the prevention and treatment of gout flare-ups. Some simple tweaks in your diet to treat gout may also reduce your risk for chronic diseases such as heart disease, obesity, and cancer. While diet is not a cure for gout, it is an adjunct therapy that may be helpful. I have counseled many clients on how to manage their gout and overall health without seeing diet changes as punishment and have seen patients experience fewer flare-ups. I'm excited to share my knowledge with you.

The Healing Gout Cookbook is a guide to sound nutrition science plus simple, delicious recipes that reduce gout flare-ups. This cookbook will help you separate fact from fiction when it comes to healthy eating. Recipes are based on both the Dietary Approaches to Stop Hypertension (DASH) diet and an anti-inflammatory diet, both of which reduce the risk of high blood pressure, heart disease, cancer, and other chronic illnesses.

In this book, you'll learn about which foods are truly "gout-friendly" and which to limit in your diet. *The Healing Gout Cookbook* will expand your understanding of uric acid and how to control your levels. You will discover which purine-containing foods will likely cause a gout flare-up and which are fairly safe to eat in moderation. As a dietitian, I want to go beyond saying what you *can't* eat and focus instead on what you *can* eat.

The recipes in this book are easy to follow and can be prepared in a short amount of time. You'll spend less time in the kitchen and enjoy more time doing the things you love without pain.

—Lisa Cicciarello Andrews, MEd, RD, LD

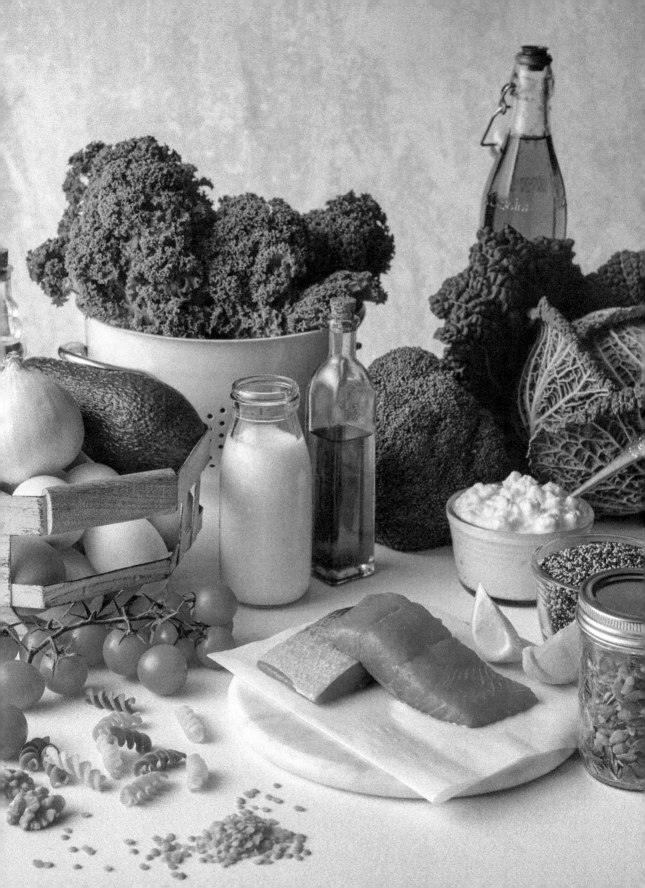

The Gout–Diet Connection

If you suffer from gout or live with someone who does, you recognize how difficult it can be to deal with. While the Internet and well-meaning friends and family are full of suggestions for how to manage the condition, information on diet and lifestyle is often conflicting. How do you know what information is true or anecdotal? This chapter will cut through the fog so you understand what it means to live with gout, learn how to fight flare-ups, and get clear on which foods are truly gout-friendly.

What Is Gout?

Gout is a painful form of arthritis that may present as acute or chronic swelling in the hands or feet. It has historically been considered "the disease of kings." Gout was first discovered by the Egyptians in 2640 BC and was thought to be triggered by the excessive consumption of rich foods and alcohol that only the wealthy could afford. The word *gout* comes from the Latin word *gutta* ("drop"). It relates to the perpetuating belief in the four "humors," an ancient Greek medical term for the liquids that they believed influenced health: blood, phlegm, yellow bile, and black bile. When in balance, the humors would maintain good health, but under certain conditions, they could move, or "drop," into a joint, creating inflammation and pain. In some eras, gout was seen as desirable by the politically and socially powerful because it implied having money to spend on fine food and wine.

Medical professionals have been treating gout for centuries. While the majority of gout patients are men between the ages of 30 and 50, women are also susceptible to gout, particularly after menopause. The risk for developing gout is based on two main factors: genetic makeup and an excess of uric acid production in the blood from the foods we eat. While we can't alter our genetic makeup, we can manage the types of foods we eat and make conscious decisions that will help prevent flare-ups. Uric acid is produced when the body breaks down purines. When uric acid levels remain high, uric acid crystals form, and the excess buildup of crystals causes painful inflammation in the joints. Purines are found in certain types of fish and other seafood, meat (beef/pork), some beans, and alcohol (especially beer).

Hyperuricemia

Hyperuricemia is the name for elevated uric acid levels in the blood, which can lead to crystal formation in joints and a potential gout attack. A normal blood level is 2.46 to 6.0 mg/dL for women and 3.4 to 7.0 mg/dL for men.

Fortunately, not everyone who has hyperuricemia will develop gout, and some people who *do* have gout don't even develop symptoms. Hyperuricemia can result from your body either creating too much uric acid or being unable to get rid of enough of it. If your kidneys are overworked removing uric acid, they may decline in function. Uric acid crystals can form anywhere in the body, but they tend to concentrate in the joints or kidneys. Drinking enough liquid, especially water, helps you filter excess uric acid out of your body.

The Stages of Gout

Like other chronic conditions, gout may progress from having little to no symptoms with no need for medication or treatment to full-blown chronic pain and inflammation. There are four stages of gout.

Stage 1 gout is known as asymptomatic gout, which means gout with no symptoms. A person may have a high level of uric acid in their blood but show no signs or symptoms of the disease. Elevated levels of uric acid may be caused by an excess intake of purines and/or a reduction in the excretion of purines.

Stage 2 gout is known as acute gouty arthritis. It also occurs due to elevated uric acid levels but is *not* pain-free. The person suffering stage 2 gout may experience sudden pain, possibly in the middle of the night. Up to 60 percent of people who have had one attack may have another gout attack within a year after their first. A diet low in purines is advised.

Stage 3 gout is known as interval gout, which means it's not quite gone but not chronic either. Stage 3 may be exacerbated by dehydration or the consumption of excess purines (often too much alcohol or excessive fatty meat or seafood intake). Diet and medication are part of treatment at this stage.

Stage 4 gout is known as chronic gout. This occurs in individuals whose uric acid levels remain elevated over a period of time, which may be related to poor kidney function, diabetes, or other conditions, including obesity. A diet low in purines with adequate fluid consumption may aid in reducing symptoms of chronic gout. Medication is likely taken on a regular basis at this phase. Medications for gout may help reduce the production or excretion of uric acid, while others may be needed for treatment of pain and inflammation.

FIGHTING FLARES

If you're dealing with an acute gout attack, there are a few things you can do to calm the inflammation and pain.

- Start by taking an anti-inflammatory medicine such as Aleve or Advil. Make sure to take with food to protect your stomach, and always check the warning labels to confirm it's safe for you.
- Drink more water to help reduce the uric acid levels in your blood. Aim for two (16 ounces total) glasses of plain water with each meal and 8 to 12 ounces in between meals. Aim for at least 8 to 16 (8-ounce) glasses daily.
- Rest, ice, and elevate the joint. This is not the time to go jogging.
- Try to reduce stress, if you're able, as it may worsen your symptoms.
- Reduce your intake of foods and drinks that increase uric acid levels. These include alcohol, red meat, and seafood high in purines.
- Reduce fried foods and high-fat sweets that may increase inflammation.

How Food Can Help

The phrase "food as medicine" has been around for years and still applies today. Not only does a healthy, nutritious diet give people the energy they need to manage their gout symptoms, but it may also help reduce the pain and inflammation of those symptoms as well as the frequency of the attacks.

Lowering Uric Acid Levels

Because high uric acid levels have been directly linked to gout attacks, it's important to find healthy ways to reduce them. Lowering uric acid levels can be achieved through diet and medication (we'll discuss medication further on page 8). It's best to avoid foods with purines, as they produce uric acid.

These foods include certain types of fish, shellfish, meat (beef/pork), some beans, and alcohol (especially beer). Alcohol in general raises uric acid levels, but beer in particular is high in purines. Wild game should also be avoided, as should yeast-containing supplements (like nutritional or brewer's yeast). Inflammatory foods that may exacerbate gout flare-ups include fried foods, fast food, high-sugar or processed desserts and beverages, and processed meats such as bacon, ham, sausage, bologna, hot dogs, and other deli meats.

On the other hand, leafy green vegetables such as spinach and kale and other vegetables may *reduce* inflammation and actually lower uric acid levels. Adding delicious cherries to your diet has also been found to reduce uric acid levels and prevent gout. (For a complete list of foods to avoid and enjoy, see pages 12–14.)

Adhering to the following guidelines will help you lower uric acid levels and reduce the risk of future gout flare-ups.

LOW-PURINE FOODS

Foods can be classified as high, medium, or low in purines. According to the American College of Rheumatology's Guidelines for Management of Gout, low-purine foods should be encouraged in patients suffering from gout. Portion size, however, is still important for weight control and blood sugar management. Low-purine foods include low-fat dairy products, whole grains, rice, pasta, and potatoes. According to the Arthritis Foundation, calcium from low-fat dairy products also helps reduce uric acid levels.

While fruit is low in purines, it does still contain sugar in the form of fructose, which you may want to limit (see the next section for more details). Nuts, seeds, and peanut butter are low in purines and contain healthy, anti-inflammatory fats. Although some vegetables such as asparagus, spinach, and cauliflower may contain purines, studies show that vegetable sources of purines do not impact gout. In fact, their anti-inflammatory properties are beneficial and should be incorporated into your daily diet.

CUT DOWN FRUCTOSE

A 2017 study published in *Nutrients* reveals a link between fructose intake and gout. Fructose (from honey, high-fructose corn syrup, fruit juice, and fruit) may increase uric acid levels, thus triggering gout flare-ups. In particular, drinking regular soda and/or consuming foods that contain high-fructose corn syrup should be avoided because they have been found to raise uric acid levels. In addition to helping control gout symptoms, limiting these beverages and foods will help with weight control and reduce the risk for cardiovascular disease and diabetes.

While you may want to limit fruit during a flare-up to avoid exacerbating your symptoms, you don't have to cut out fruit entirely. Instead, choose fruit in its whole form for its fiber and other phytochemicals that help reduce inflammation.

THE BENEFITS OF ANTIOXIDANTS

Antioxidants are helpful compounds that come from fruits, vegetables, whole grains, nuts, seeds, and beans. They have been found to reduce the risk of chronic diseases such as cancer and heart disease by protecting cells within the body. Plant chemicals, known as "phytochemicals," help reduce inflammation, which can help protect your cells from damage. Dark orange fruits and vegetables contain vitamin C and beta-carotene, the phytochemical that gives carrots and sweet potatoes their bright orange color. Berries, cherries, citrus fruit, melon, and other fruits are high in vitamin C and other antioxidants, as are green leafy vegetables and tomatoes. Other foods that contain antioxidants include those high in vitamin E, such as nuts, seeds, and healthy oils from plants such as canola, corn, and olive oil. Whole grains such as whole-wheat bread, quinoa, bulgur, and farro are also sources of antioxidants such as selenium and vitamin E. Finally, resveratrol is a type of antioxidant that is found in dark red, purple, or black grapes; grape juice; peanuts; pistachios; blueberries; cocoa; and red wine.

STAY HYDRATED

Drinking enough water and other fluids is vital to staying hydrated and preventing gout attacks. Water helps filter waste products from your kidneys, including excess uric acid. Decaffeinated coffee, tea, or sugar-free drinks can also help keep you hydrated. Also keep in mind that fruits, vegetables, and low-sodium broth-based soups also contain plenty of fluids. Signs of dehydration include dark urine, dry mouth, or feeling "woozy" when you stand up.

MEDICATIONS

There are multiple medications that can be used to treat gout by reducing uric acid production, reducing uric acid levels in the blood, or helping relieve pain and inflammation during a flare-up. Always discuss which medication is right for you with your doctor or pharmacist. The following are some commonly prescribed and over-the-counter (OTC) medications.

- **Allopurinol** and **Febuxostat** reduce uric acid production.
- **Colchicine** reduces inflammation.
- **Lesinurad** helps you eliminate uric acid through urine.
- **Pegloticase** breaks down uric acid.
- **Probenecid** works in your kidneys to get rid of uric acid.

- **Indomethacin** is a prescription non-steroidal, anti-inflammatory (NSAID) pain reliever, while Aleve (naproxen) and Advil (ibuprofen) are over-the-counter NSAIDs.
- **Steroids** (aka corticosteroids) are prescription medications that help reduce inflammation. These include **prednisone**, **dexamethasone**, and **methylprednisolone**.

Recent research has linked diuretics, sometimes known as "water pills," with increased uric acid levels, which may raise your risk for gout attacks. Diuretics are medications such as Lasix or hydrochlorothiazide that are often prescribed for people with high blood pressure, congestive heart failure, or other conditions in which the body retains too much sodium or fluid. Your doctor can discuss side effects of these medications with you.

Some questions you can ask your doctor include:

1. Which medication is right for me? How long will I need to take it?
2. How soon will this medicine relieve my pain?
3. What are common side effects of my medication?

Comorbid Diseases

Individuals dealing with gout may often be dealing with other chronic illnesses or be at risk for developing them. Eating foods low in purines and high in antioxidants may help reduce your risk of other diseases. Look at it like killing two (or three) birds with one stone!

When uric acid levels increase in the blood, your kidneys must work harder, increasing the potential for kidney disease. Reducing sodium intake from canned, frozen, processed, and fast foods will help keep your blood pressure in check and reduce this risk. Staying hydrated and getting *moderate* amounts of protein from dairy products, meat, fish, poultry, and vegetable sources such as beans, nuts, soy-based products, and seeds will also keep your kidneys from having to work too hard.

A gout-friendly diet may also reduce the risk for heart disease. When you reduce your intake of fatty cuts of meat, fried foods, full-fat dairy products, and high-sugar foods, you are doing your heart a big favor, since those foods tend to increase cholesterol and blood sugar levels. Focusing instead on a plant-based diet with lots of fruits and vegetables as well as whole grains, beans, nuts, and healthy fats has been shown to reduce heart disease. The American Heart Association also advises two or more servings of fish per week to reduce the risk of heart disease. Salmon, for example, is low in purines and high in omega-3 fatty acids (and you'll find multiple recipes for it in this book).

As obesity rates in the United States increase, diabetes has become more common. A diet lower in added sugar from soda, high-calorie desserts, candy, and other processed carbs can help keep weight in check while also reducing the risk for gout. Carrying excess weight reduces the body's ability to get rid of uric acid, making obesity a contributing factor in the onset of gout. Regular exercise improves insulin sensitivity (the body's ability to use insulin), aids in weight management, and may help reduce inflammation when gout flare-ups occur. To help manage weight, you should aim for a body mass index (BMI) between 19 and 25.

Related Diets

As is the case with other chronic conditions, improving eating habits can help manage people's gout. The Dietary Guidelines for Americans—which are updated every five years as nutrition science evolves—may be a helpful guide for those dealing with gout, as they recommend a diet that is lower in saturated fat, sugar, and sodium and higher in plant-based foods, lean protein sources, and low-fat dairy products. Gout-friendly eating combines aspects of the following healthy diets.

Anti-Inflammatory Diet

Since gout flare-ups involve inflammation of the joints, it can be helpful to limit inflammatory foods while consuming foods that reduce inflammation. High-fat, animal-based foods such as fatty cuts of beef and pork, full-fat dairy products, fried and fast foods, and high-sugar desserts tend to be more inflammatory. Overeating also impacts the immune system, which may trigger the body to produce inflammatory chemicals.

An anti-inflammatory diet, on the other hand, is plant-based, consisting of lots of vegetables, fruits, beans and legumes, nuts and seeds, low-fat dairy products, lean meat, and whole-grain breads, cereals, and other grains.

Beverages like green and black tea and coffee may also help reduce inflammation. Certain spices such as turmeric and cinnamon add not only a kick but also anti-inflammatory properties to foods.

DASH Diet

DASH stands for Dietary Approaches to Stop Hypertension. This diet was developed by the National Heart, Lung, and Blood Institute to help reduce high blood pressure. What's interesting is that this diet has also been found to reduce the risk for diabetes and heart disease. The DASH diet is similar to the anti-inflammatory diet in that it also emphasizes fruits, vegetables, whole grains, low-fat dairy products, and lean or low-fat animal foods while limiting sodium, saturated fat, cholesterol, sugar, and high-fat animal foods. Because gout patients are at risk for heart disease, it may be especially important to follow a heart-healthy diet.

The old saying "you are what you eat" couldn't be truer. While it's important to enjoy food, it's equally important to think of food as a source of energy and nutrition and explore fun ways to optimize the benefits of food. Following the anti-inflammatory diet or the DASH diet is beneficial for long-term health because what we eat either prevents or promotes disease. Managing blood pressure and blood sugar reduces your risk for heart disease and stroke as well as kidney disease. Research indicates that populations with diets high in plant-based foods have the lowest rates of chronic diseases, including obesity, heart disease, cancer, diabetes, and arthritis—all good reasons to eat a nutritious diet!

Managing Gout WHAT TO EAT AT A GLANCE

Dealing with gout is a balancing act. Some foods may increase uric acid production and inflammation and should be avoided as much as possible, while others will reduce inflammation and promote healing and should be eaten more frequently. The key is to have fun, be smart, and choose the right foods.

FOODS TO AVOID

DAIRY (FULL-FAT)

- Cheese
- Cream cheese
- Full-fat yogurt
- Sour cream
- Premium ice cream
- Whole milk

DRINKS

- Beer
- Drinks containing high-fructose corn syrup (soda, sports drinks)
- Fruit juices containing added sugar or corn syrup
- Liquor

FISH/SEAFOOD

- Anchovies
- Codfish
- Haddock
- Herring
- Mackerel
- Mussels
- Perch
- Sardines
- Scallops
- Trout
- Tuna

GRAINS

- Sweetened cereal
- Donuts and other pastries, full-fat ice cream

MEATS

- Bacon
- High-fat cuts of beef (burgers, ribeye steaks, T-bone steak)
- High-fat cuts of pork (pork chops, pork ribs, pork shoulder)
- High-fat lunch meat (bologna, pickle loaf, roast beef)
- Lamb
- Organ meats (brains, kidney, liver, sweetbreads [thymus gland or pancreas])
- Processed meats (hot dogs, bacon, sausage)
- Wild game (duck, goose, venison)

OTHERS

- Mung beans
- Yeast extract (Marmite) and brewer's yeast (a nutritional supplement)

FOODS TO EAT IN MODERATION

DRINKS

- 100% fruit juice
- Wine

FATS

- Butter
- Coconut oil
- Margarine
- Vegetable oil
- Wheat germ oil

FISH/SEAFOOD

- Crab
- Lobster
- Oysters
- Shrimp

GRAINS

- Oats and oatmeal
- Saltines and other crackers
- Wheat bran

OTHERS

- Candy
- Chocolate
- Fava beans
- Chickpeas

MEATS

- Chicken
- Ham
- Lean cuts of red meat and pork (flank steak, sirloin, tenderloin)
- Turkey

FOODS TO ENCOURAGE

DAIRY

- Eggs
- Egg substitutes
- Low-fat cheese
- Low-fat cottage cheese
- Low-fat yogurt
- Skim or 1% milk

DRINKS

- Coffee
- Tea
- Seltzer
- Water

FATS

- Canola oil
- Corn oil
- Grapeseed oil
- Olive oil
- Peanut oil
- Sesame oil
- Walnut oil

FISH/SEAFOOD

- Catfish
- Flounder
- Red snapper
- Salmon
- Sea bass
- Sole
- Swai (aka basa)
- Tilapia
- Whitefish

FRUITS
- Apples
- Apricots
- Avocados
- Bananas
- Berries (blackberries, blueberries, raspberries, strawberries)
- Cherries
- Citrus fruits (grapefruit, oranges, mandarins, tangerines)
- Grapes
- Kiwi
- Melon (cantaloupe, honeydew, watermelon)
- Nectarines
- Peaches
- Pears
- Raisins
- Prunes

GRAINS
- Barley
- Bread
- Bulgur
- Farro
- Pasta
- Popcorn
- Pretzels
- Quinoa
- Rice
- Unsweetened cereals
- Wheat
- Whole-grain cereals and crackers

OTHER
- Broth-based soups
- Almond butter
- Gelatin
- Lentils
- Nuts (any)
- Peanut butter
- Seeds (chia, flaxseeds, pumpkin, sunflower)

VEGETABLES
- Asparagus
- Broccoli
- Brussels sprouts
- Cabbage
- Carrots
- Cauliflower
- Collard greens
- Corn
- Green beans
- Eggplant
- Kale
- Kohlrabi
- Lettuce
- Mushrooms
- Radishes
- Potatoes
- Spinach
- Sweet potatoes
- Tomatoes
- Wax beans

Your Flare-Free Kitchen

Stocking your kitchen with nutritious foods that are low in purines will help you easily follow a gout-friendly diet. Replacing processed foods with nutrient-dense fruits, vegetables, whole grains, lean protein sources, and low-fat dairy products will also help control uric acid levels in the long run.

You may be sharing a kitchen with others who likely do not need to follow a gout-friendly diet. It may be helpful to organize your kitchen so that a cupboard or section of the refrigerator is sectioned off for your gout-friendly foods. Ask family or friends to help support your efforts by keeping trigger foods out of your space.

A gout-friendly diet does not have to be difficult or expensive to follow; it just takes a conscious effort to make the best choices. It's something you can have fun with! The following are lists of healthy foods to keep stocked in your kitchen. Remember, shopping for seasonal produce and choosing water over alcohol and sugary drinks can help keep expenses down. Try to avoid foods with a lot of added sugars (more than 10 grams per serving) or that are high in sodium (more than 300 mg per serving).

Pantry Essentials

DRINKS
- Coffee
- Tea
- Water (Consider a time-stamped water bottle to help you drink enough through-out the day.)

FATS
- Canola oil
- Corn oil
- Olive oil
- Peanut oil

FRUIT
- Canned fruit packed in water or 100% juice
- Dried fruit (any kind)
- Individual fruit cups packed in water or 100% juice

GRAINS

- Bagged or boxed grains (barley, bulgur, couscous, pasta, quinoa, rice, etc.)
- Crackers
- Popcorn
- Pretzels
- Unsweetened cereal

OTHER

- Beef or chicken broth (low-sodium)
- Dried herbs
- Spices
- Vinegar

PROTEIN SOURCES

- Almond or peanut butter
- Canned or bagged beans
- Canned chicken
- Lentils
- Nuts (any kind)

VEGETABLES

- Canned vegetables (no-salt), including carrots, corn, green beans, mixed vegetables, and tomatoes
- Individual packs of vegetables
- Low-sodium vegetable juice

Fridge and Freezer Essentials

CONDIMENTS

- Ginger paste
- Ketchup
- Low-sodium soy sauce
- Minced garlic
- Mustards (brown, Dijon, yellow, etc.)

DAIRY

- Eggs, egg whites
- Low-fat cheese
- Low-fat or nonfat yogurt
- Skim or 1% milk

DRINKS

- 100% fruit juice, especially tart cherry juice
- Seltzer
- Unsweetened iced tea
- Water

FROZEN ITEMS

- Frozen brown rice
- Frozen fish
- Frozen fruit
- Frozen poultry
- Frozen vegetables
- Frozen veggie burgers
- Frozen whole-grain waffles

FRUITS

- Any fresh fruits, particularly dark cherries, but also apples, bananas, grapes, kiwis, melons, nectarines, peaches, pears, and pineapples

VEGETABLES

- Any fresh vegetables, including broccoli, Brussels sprouts, carrots, cauliflower, green beans, kale, and spinach

Cooking Equipment

Having the right cooking equipment can motivate and encourage you to prepare your own meals and rely less on fast or processed foods. While you can make do without some of the following items, they'll make your life in the kitchen a lot easier—and faster. You don't have to be a gourmet chef to make delicious, gout-friendly meals, and these tools can help.

ESSENTIALS

- Aluminum foil
- Bakeware (9-by-13-inch and 8-by-8-inch pans, muffin tins)
- Broiler pan
- Can opener
- Colander
- Cutting boards
- Hand mixer
- Knives
- Measuring cups and spoons
- Mixing bowls
- Parchment paper
- Sauce pans (small, medium, and large)
- Serving spoons/forks
- Sheet pans
- Skillets (medium and large)
- Slow cooker
- Vegetable peeler
- Whisks
- Wooden spoons

NICE TO HAVES

- Blender
- Citrus juicer
- Coffeepot
- Egg separator
- Food processor
- Grater
- Grill pan
- Indoor grill (e.g., George Foreman Grill)
- Instant Pot
- Kitchen scale
- Knife sharpener
- Ladles
- Meat thermometer
- Rice cooker
- Salad spinner
- Stand mixer
- Stockpot
- Toaster oven
- Trivets
- Zester

OUTSIDE YOUR OWN KITCHEN

Although your kitchen may be well stocked and ready for action, there will certainly be times when you'd rather eat out or are eating in someone else's home. Dealing with gout flare-ups is not following a fad diet for a few months; it's a lifestyle choice and a complete shift. Even when you're not cooking, it's important to keep an eye on what you eat to prevent the chance of flare-ups.

By learning which foods may trigger a gout attack, you'll be better equipped to know what to eat and what to avoid or limit in your diet. There are plenty of tasty foods that are low in purines and won't trigger a flare-up.

When eating out, consider heart-healthy choices. Limit beef, fatty cuts of meat, and high-sugar and high-fat desserts such as cake, ice cream, cheesecake, and other pastries. Choose broth-based soups and tomato-based pastas instead of dishes served in heavy cream or cheese. Add more vegetables to your plate by ordering a salad or requesting an extra side of veggies. Drink water, coffee, or tea in place of sweetened soda, iced tea, or alcohol.

Special occasions such as birthdays, holidays, and parties don't have to be difficult. You can bring seltzer water if you're trying to avoid alcohol, or you can offer to bring a veggie or fruit tray as an appetizer. Having a snack before the event may keep you from overindulging or eating something that may cause a flare-up.

Being on vacation is a time of relaxation and fun but may be challenging if you're trying to manage what you eat. You can stick to your gout-friendly diet by looking up a restaurant's menu ahead of time and paying attention to the ingredients listed in each dish so you can tell which foods will be safest to eat.

About the Recipes

As a dietitian, giving you information about what you *can* eat will help more than just telling you what you *can't* eat. The recipes in this book will focus on delicious meals that should help prevent flare-ups. They're designed to minimize high-purine foods, saturated fat, sugar, and sodium while providing variety and flavor.

This book's recipes are based on ingredients that are seasonal, easy to find, and simple to prepare. You and your family will be eating nutritious food so delicious, I promise you that it won't feel like you're "on a diet."

All of the recipes contained in this book are heart-healthy, low in purines, or anti-inflammatory—or all three! For example, Dillicious Fish with Roasted Broccoli (page 66) is low in fat and a good source of potassium, making it heart-healthy, anti-inflammatory, *and* low in purines.

Each recipe will be labeled for dietary restrictions.

- **Kidney-friendly** recipes will have less than 350mg of sodium and less than 200mg of potassium per serving.
- **Diabetic-friendly** recipes will have less than 8 grams of added sugars and less than 35 grams of total of carbohydrates per serving.
- **Vegan** recipes will be completely plant-based and without animal products of any kind, such as dairy, eggs, fish, or meat.
- **Vegetarian** recipes are plant-based without meat or fish but may contain eggs or dairy products.
- **Gluten-free** recipes will not contain barley, oats, rye, or wheat. They are suitable for those following a gluten-free diet, but you should always check your ingredients for gluten-free labels.
- **30-minute** recipes will take 30 minutes or less including prep and cook time.
- **One-pot** recipes use only one main pot or pan, not including bowls.

Each recipe will also provide a helpful tip to either modify the recipe or offer an optional step to make your life easier. These include cooking tips to explain or simplify the process, variation tips to change things up or make use of leftovers, substitution tips to swap out ingredients, and trigger tips to optimize recipes according to your individual needs.

ALMOND OATMEAL PANCAKES

29

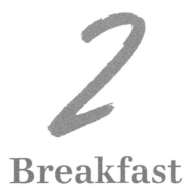

Breakfast

This chapter will help you start out every day on the right, gout-free foot. It includes both sweet and savory dishes such as Turkey Sausage Patty Melt with Spinach (page 26), Avocado and Black Bean Toast with Spicy Salsa (page 31), and Orange Cinnamon French Toast with Maple Syrup (page 30). You'll find both vegetarian and non-vegetarian recipe options throughout.

GREEN EGGS, NO PAN

SERVES 1 **PREP TIME** 2 MINUTES **COOK TIME** 3 MINUTES

Looking for a fast egg recipe that includes all the important nutrients to kick-start your day? In this dish, eggs aren't boiled or boring. They can be cooked in a microwave with any number of veggies for a quick, satisfying breakfast. Spinach, peppers, or tomatoes provide a healthy dose of vitamin C, an anti-inflammatory antioxidant. If you're looking to feed more, you can easily double or triple the recipe.

✓ **DIABETIC FRIENDLY**

✓ **ONE POT**

✓ **VEGETARIAN**

Nonstick cooking spray

1 egg

1 teaspoon water

1 cup fresh spinach leaves or other chopped veggies (onions, peppers, tomatoes, mushrooms, etc.)

½ teaspoon oregano

1 whole-wheat English muffin (optional)

1 teaspoon shredded Cheddar cheese

Salt

Freshly ground black pepper

1. Spray the inside of a small, microwave-safe bowl with nonstick spray. Crack the egg into the bowl, add the water, and scramble the egg with a fork or whisk.

2. Add spinach and oregano on top of the egg and microwave for 1 minute.

3. While the egg is cooking, toast an English muffin, if desired.

4. Remove the egg from the microwave and sprinkle cheese over the spinach. Microwave for 20 to 30 seconds, or until the cheese is melted. Season with salt and pepper as desired.

5. Take the English muffin out of the toaster (if using) and place it on a plate. Fold the egg in half and place on the bottom half of the muffin; then place the top half on top to make a sandwich.

SUBSTITUTION TIP: Try roasted peppers or cooked zucchini instead of spinach.

PER SERVING: Total Calories: 82; Total Fat: 5g; Saturated Fat: 2g; Cholesterol: 166mg; Sodium: 100mg; Potassium: 241mg; Total Carbohydrate: 2g; Fiber: 1g; Sugars: 1g; Protein: 7g

GINGER AND CINNAMON BREAKFAST QUINOA

SERVES 4 **PREP TIME** 5 MINUTES **COOK TIME** 15 MINUTES

Quinoa is known as a gluten-free "ancient grain" that originates from Peru. It's higher in protein and fiber than other grains, which means it promotes fullness. It's also a decent source of iron—a nutrient people are often deficient in, particularly women and children. Quinoa also can be used in savory dishes with vegetables and beans.

✓ 30-MINUTE

✓ GLUTEN-FREE

✓ ONE POT

✓ VEGAN

2 cups water

1 cup dry quinoa

1 teaspoon brown sugar

1 teaspoon ginger paste

½ teaspoon
  ground cinnamon

½ teaspoon vanilla extract

1 tablespoon
  chopped pecans

1 tablespoon raisins

1. Place the water and quinoa in a medium pan and bring to a boil. Cook for 5 minutes; then turn the heat down and simmer for 12 to 14 minutes, or until the quinoa is soft and all the water has been absorbed.

2. While the quinoa is hot, mix in the brown sugar, ginger paste, cinnamon, vanilla, pecans, and raisins. Serve warm.

VARIATION TIP: You can add chopped apples or dried fruit such as apricots to the quinoa to make it even more filling.

PER SERVING: Total Calories: 220; Total Fat: 8g; Saturated Fat: 1g; Cholesterol: 0mg; Sodium: 14mg; Potassium: 288mg; Total Carbohydrate: 41g; Fiber: 4g; Sugars: 2g; Protein: 7g

BERRY BREAKFAST YOGURT PARFAIT

SERVES 2   **PREP TIME** 5 MINUTES

This recipe is so simple but so delicious you'll feel like you're having dessert for breakfast. It combines DASH-friendly yogurt (a good source of calcium and vitamin D for bone and heart health) with antioxidant-rich berries, chopped walnuts, and ground flaxseed. It can be made ahead of time and ready by morning or assembled right before eating.

✓ **30-MINUTE**
✓ **DIABETIC FRIENDLY**
✓ **GLUTEN-FREE**
✓ **KIDNEY FRIENDLY**
✓ **ONE POT**
✓ **VEGETARIAN**

2 cups plain, low-fat Greek yogurt

1 cup fresh or frozen berries (blueberries, strawberries, raspberries, or a mix)

4 tablespoons ground flaxseed

½ cup chopped walnuts

1. Using two 8- to 12-ounce mason jars or clear glasses, layer ½ cup of Greek yogurt on the bottom of each. Top the yogurt with ¼ cup of berries of choice. Add 1 tablespoon of ground flaxseed over the berries.

2. Layer another ½ cup of Greek yogurt over the berries. Add the remaining ¼ cup of berries over the Greek yogurt. Top the berries with another tablespoon of ground flaxseed.

3. Add ¼ cup chopped walnuts to each jar.

SUBSTITUTION TIP: If you don't have berries, you can use chopped pears and cinnamon instead.

PER SERVING: Total Calories: 469; Total Fat: 26g; Saturated Fat: 3g; Cholesterol: 6mg; Sodium: 127mg; Potassium: 90mg; Total Carbohydrate: 27g; Fiber: 8g; Sugars: 16g; Protein: 34g

PEANUT BUTTER AND BANANA BREAKFAST WRAP

SERVES 2 **PREP TIME** 5 MINUTES

It's no wonder Elvis loved the combination of peanut butter and bananas—they are simply delicious together! This easy breakfast wrap is a good source of dietary fiber as well as potassium, which helps lower blood pressure. It can be made ahead of time and even cut into fun "wheelies" for kids.

✓ **30-MINUTE**

✓ **ONE POT**

✓ **VEGAN**

2 medium (10-inch) whole-wheat tortillas

4 tablespoons smooth or crunchy peanut butter

1 banana, cut into ½-inch slices

1 teaspoon honey

1 tablespoon chia seeds, divided

1. Place the whole-wheat tortillas on plates and spread 2 tablespoons of peanut butter on each. Top the peanut butter with banana slices and drizzle ½ teaspoon of honey over the bananas.

2. Sprinkle ½ tablespoon of chia seeds over the honey on each tortilla.

3. Roll the tortillas up and serve or refrigerate for up to 24 hours.

SUBSTITUTION TIP: To make this recipe kidney friendly, used chopped apples instead of bananas.

PER SERVING: Total Calories: 453; Total Fat: 22g; Saturated Fat: 4g; Cholesterol: 0mg; Sodium: 689mg; Potassium: 450mg; Total Carbohydrate: 61g; Fiber: 12g; Sugars: 13g; Protein: 17g

TURKEY SAUSAGE PATTY MELT WITH SPINACH

SERVES 2   **PREP TIME** 5 MINUTES   **COOK TIME** 10 MINUTES

If you're a fan of sausage but don't want all the saturated fat, try turkey sausage. This tasty breakfast sandwich combines savory turkey sausage with Swiss cheese and anti-inflammatory spinach. It is served on toasted rye bread, which has been found to curb appetite. If you'd like to boost the protein content, add a scrambled or fried egg.

✓ **30-MINUTE**
✓ **DIABETIC FRIENDLY**
✓ **ONE POT**

2 turkey sausage patties
2 slices rye bread
10 fresh spinach leaves
2 slices Swiss cheese

1. In a small skillet, cook the turkey sausage patties for 4 to 6 minutes per side, or until fully cooked.

2. Meanwhile, toast the rye bread in a toaster or toaster oven.

3. Once the patties are done, place 5 spinach leaves and a slice of Swiss cheese on each patty. Place a lid on the skillet for 2 minutes to wilt the spinach and melt the cheese.

4. Cut the slices of rye bread in half. Place one sausage patty on one half-slice of the bread and top with another half-slice. Repeat to make the second sandwich.

SUBSTITUTION TIP: You can use whole-wheat or any other whole-grain bread instead of rye bread.

TRIGGER TIP: If turkey tends to trigger a flare-up, you can use vegetarian breakfast patties instead of turkey sausage.

PER SERVING: Total Calories: 298; Total Fat: 14g; Saturated Fat: 6g; Cholesterol: 66mg; Sodium: 813mg; Potassium: 301mg; Total Carbohydrate: 22g; Fiber: 2g; Sugars: 1g; Protein: 23g

BLACK BEAN BREAKFAST SCRAMBLE

SERVES 2   **PREP TIME** 7 MINUTES   **COOK TIME** 10 MINUTES

If you need a quick breakfast to fill you up and tickle your taste buds, look no further. This delicious breakfast scramble combines fluffy scrambled eggs with high-fiber black beans, onions, and salsa. This scramble is a great source of protein and can be eaten on its own or served with a bowl of fresh fruit.

✓ **30-MINUTE**
✓ **DIABETIC FRIENDLY**
✓ **GLUTEN-FREE**
✓ **ONE POT**
✓ **VEGETARIAN**

4 large eggs

4 teaspoons water

1 teaspoon ground cumin

½ cup canned black beans, drained and rinsed

2 tablespoons chopped onions

1 tablespoon corn oil or olive oil

2 tablespoons prepared salsa

¼ cup shredded Cheddar cheese

2 tablespoons chopped green onions (green and white parts)

1. Combine the eggs, water, and cumin in a large mixing bowl and whisk together. Stir in the black beans and onions.

2. In a nonstick skillet, heat the oil and add the egg mixture. Scramble until fully cooked, about five minutes.

3. Remove the egg mixture from the pan and place on a plate. Top with salsa, Cheddar cheese, and green onions.

COOKING TIP: For a faster prep time, you can make this dish in the microwave. Combine the eggs, water, cumin, onions, and black beans in a microwave-safe bowl. Heat the mixture for 2 to 4 minutes, or until eggs are fully cooked. Once cooked, place on a plate, add the salsa, Cheddar cheese, and green onions.

PER SERVING: Total Calories: 331; Total Fat: 22g; Saturated Fat: 7g; Cholesterol: 387mg; Sodium: 327mg; Potassium: 398mg; Total Carbohydrate: 14g; Fiber: 5g; Sugars: 2g; Protein: 21g

PEPPER AND ONION BREAKFAST MUFFINS

SERVES 4   **PREP TIME** 5 MINUTES   **COOK TIME** 25 MINUTES

This is one of the most versatile breakfast recipes around. These muffins can be made ahead of time and are great for breakfast, an afternoon snack, or even a simple dinner. Eggs provide a gout-friendly, protein-rich meal that can easily be paired with veggies and savory spices. Enjoy these muffins with whole-grain toast or your favorite breakfast bread.

✓ **30-MINUTE**
✓ **DIABETIC FRIENDLY**
✓ **GLUTEN-FREE**
✓ **ONE POT**
✓ **VEGAN**

Nonstick spray

1 small red bell
 pepper, diced

1 small green bell
 pepper, diced

½ white or yellow onion,
 finely chopped

8 large eggs

¼ teaspoon seasoned salt

¼ teaspoon dried rosemary

¼ teaspoon dried oregano

1. Place a rack in the middle of the oven and preheat to 350°F. Spray a 12-cup muffin tin with nonstick spray.

2. Divide red and green bell peppers and chopped onions among the muffin cups.

3. In a large mixing bowl, whisk the eggs, seasoned salt, rosemary, and oregano together. Using a ladle, pour ¼ cup of the egg mixture into each muffin cup.

4. Bake the muffins for 23 to 25 minutes, or until eggs are set.

5. Let the muffins cool for a few minutes. Then, using a butter knife, loosen the muffins from the tin.

6. Serve the muffins while hot or refrigerate and use within 5 days. If freezing muffins, cool them completely, seal in an airtight container, and eat within 3 months.

VARIATION TIP: To change up this recipe, you can use spinach and zucchini instead of peppers and onions.

PER SERVING: Total Calories: 162; Total Fat: 10g; Saturated Fat: 3g; Cholesterol: 372mg; Sodium: 237mg; Potassium: 245mg; Total Carbohydrate: 4g; Fiber: 1g; Sugars: 3g; Protein: 13g

ALMOND OATMEAL PANCAKES

SERVES 4   **PREP TIME** 10 MINUTES   **COOK TIME** 15 MINUTES

This will be your new favorite pancake recipe! Using whole-wheat flour and oats boosts the fiber in this recipe without compromising taste. Chopped almonds add flavor and crunch and pair nicely with warm maple syrup. If you don't have buttermilk on hand, never fear: Add a tablespoon of white or apple cider vinegar to milk to curdle and sour the milk.

✓ **30-MINUTE**
✓ **KIDNEY**
✓ **ONE POT**
✓ **VEGETARIAN**

½ cup all-purpose flour

½ cup whole-wheat flour

½ cup quick oats

¼ cup chopped almonds

2 tablespoons brown sugar

2 teaspoons baking powder

2 teaspoons baking soda

½ teaspoon salt

1¼ cups buttermilk

2 eggs

¼ cup canola oil

Nonstick spray

Maple syrup or honey,
  for serving

Fresh blueberries, for
  topping (optional)

1. In a large mixing bowl, combine the all-purpose and whole-wheat flours, quick oats, chopped almonds, brown sugar, baking powder, baking soda, and salt.

2. Whisk in the buttermilk, eggs, and canola oil until just combined.

3. Preheat a griddle to medium-high heat and spray with nonstick spray.

4. Pour out ¼ cup of pancake batter onto the griddle. Cook the pancakes until bubbles form on the surface. Flip and continue cooking until golden brown.

5. Serve pancakes with maple syrup or honey. Top with blueberries, if desired.

VARIATION TIP: For more flavor, add 2 teaspoons of cinnamon to the dry ingredients.

PER SERVING: Total Calories: 394; Total Fat: 21g; Saturated Fat: 3g; Cholesterol: 85mg; Sodium: 836mg; Potassium: 564mg; Total Carbohydrate: 41g; Fiber: 4g; Sugars: 9g; Protein: 12g

ORANGE CINNAMON FRENCH TOAST WITH MAPLE SYRUP

SERVES 2   **PREP TIME** 5 MINUTES   **COOK TIME** 15 MINUTES

If you think rye bread would make strange French toast, think again. Its rustic texture and savory flavor pair nicely with sweet orange and cinnamon and provide a delightful change to this traditional recipe. Rye bread has been found to help reduce appetite and lead to better blood sugar levels than wheat bread. This recipe can be doubled or tripled for others to enjoy it.

✓ **30-MINUTE**
✓ **ONE POT**
✓ **VEGETARIAN**

2 eggs

1 teaspoon orange extract

½ teaspoon ground cinnamon

¼ cup milk

4 slices rye bread

Nonstick spray

Maple syrup, for serving

1. In a shallow mixing bowl, beat the eggs, orange extract, cinnamon, and milk. Dip the rye bread into the egg mixture, turning it to coat each side evenly.

2. Heat a griddle or skillet over medium heat and lightly grease with nonstick spray. Place the bread on the griddle and cook until browned on both sides.

3. Serve with warm maple syrup.

VARIATION TIP: To change things up, try using almond extract instead of orange.

PER SERVING: Total Calories: 348; Total Fat: 7g; Saturated Fat: 2g; Cholesterol: 166mg; Sodium: 502mg; Potassium: 266mg; Total Carbohydrate: 60g; Fiber: 4g; Sugars: 28g; Protein: 12g

AVOCADO AND BLACK BEAN TOAST WITH SPICY SALSA

SERVES 2 **PREP TIME** 5 MINUTES **COOK TIME** 5 MINUTES

If you enjoy avocado toast, this is a real treat. Avocados are popular for their creamy texture and versatility and are a great source of potassium and heart-healthy, anti-inflammatory monounsaturated fat. Combine traditional avocado toast with black beans and salsa to boost protein, fiber, and antioxidant levels.

✓ **30-MINUTE**

✓ **DIABETIC FRIENDLY**

✓ **GLUTEN-FREE**

✓ **ONE POT**

✓ **VEGAN**

½ cup canned black beans, drained and rinsed

¼ cup prepared salsa

2 slices multigrain or sourdough bread

1 avocado

Pinch salt

1. In a small bowl, combine the black beans and salsa and set aside.

2. Toast the bread until golden brown.

3. While the bread toasts, slice the avocado and remove the pit. Scoop out the avocado flesh using a small spoon and place it into a bowl. Mash the avocado with a fork, leaving it slightly chunky. Add a pinch of salt for flavor.

4. Place the toasted bread on plates. Divide the avocado between the two pieces of toast and top with the black bean mixture.

SUBSTITUTION TIP: You can use pinto beans if you don't have black beans on hand.

PER SERVING: Total Calories: 279; Total Fat: 15g; Saturated Fat: 2g; Cholesterol: 0mg; Sodium: 412mg; Potassium: 767mg; Total Carbohydrate: 31g; Fiber: 12g; Sugars: 3g; Protein: 10g

COCONUT PECAN OATMEAL WITH APPLES AND CINNAMON

SERVES 4   **PREP TIME** 5 MINUTES   **COOK TIME** 10 MINUTES

This delicious breakfast combines anti-inflammatory cherries with apples and coconut. The oats and apples provide soluble fiber to help lower cholesterol, and coconut and chopped pecans add a delightful crunchy texture. This recipe can be doubled or tripled to feed a crowd.

✓ **30-MINUTE**
✓ **ONE POT**
✓ **VEGETARIAN**

2 cups rolled oats

1 cup water

1 cup milk

2 teaspoons ground cinnamon

2 apples, cored and chopped

½ cup dried cherries

½ cup coconut flakes

½ cup pecans, chopped

1. Heat a large saucepan over medium heat. Add the oats, water, milk, and cinnamon, and stir until combined. Add the apples and cherries and bring to a boil. Cook for 3 minutes, and then reduce heat and simmer for 5 more minutes.

2. Stir in the coconut flakes and pecans and serve.

VARIATION TIP: Not a coconut fan? Leave it out. Ground flax-seed could also be added, if desired, to boost omega-3 fatty acid content.

COOKING TIP: Overnight oats can be made by combining 2 cups of rolled oats with 1 cup of milk and 1 cup of water. Add the cinnamon, apples, cherries, coconut flakes, and pecans. Stir everything together and chill overnight in the refrigerator.

PER SERVING: Total Calories: 455; Total Fat: 19g; Saturated Fat: 7g; Cholesterol: 5mg; Sodium: 35mg; Potassium: 415mg; Total Carbohydrate: 67g; Fiber: 11g; Sugars: 28g; Protein: 10g

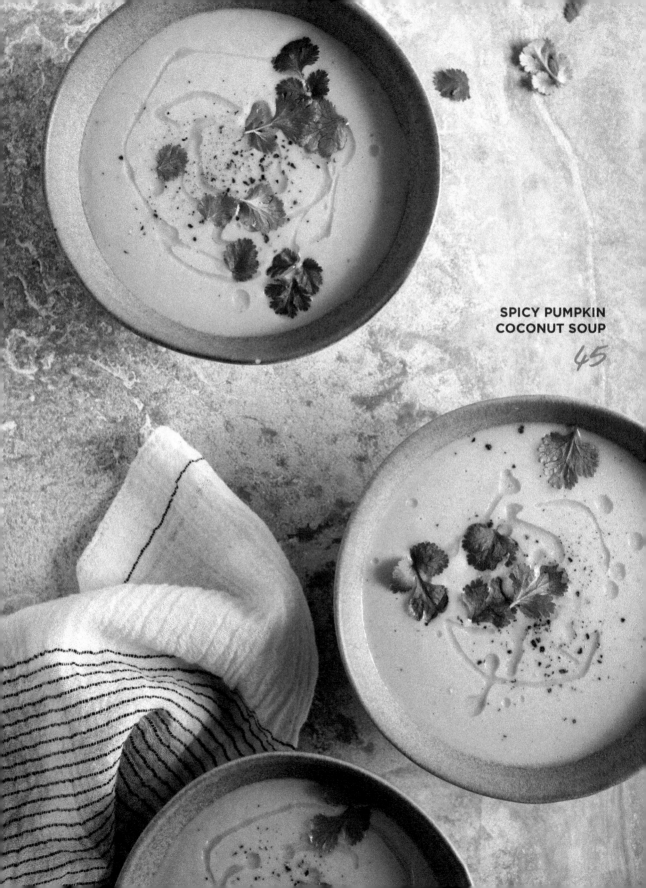

SPICY PUMPKIN
COCONUT SOUP

45

3

Soups, Salads, and Sides

This chapter has everything you need to prepare delicious, light dishes that will liven up any meal with a wide variety of tastes and textures. Think Ginger Mashed Sweet Potatoes (page 36), Kale Strawberry Salad (page 37), Fiesta Rice (page 43), and Arugula and Spinach Salad in Citrus Dressing (page 42). The recipes are so tasty, you'll forget they're healthy.

GINGER MASHED SWEET POTATOES

SERVES 6   **PREP TIME** 7 MINUTES   **COOK TIME** 35 MINUTES

Want something sweet for a holiday meal but not the traditional marshmallow-laden casserole? I've got just the recipe for you. Mashed sweet potatoes are delicious combined with ginger, cinnamon, and orange juice. They provide a hefty dose of anti-inflammatory beta-carotene and vitamin C without all the added sugar. This dish goes great with pork, chicken, or fish.

✓ **GLUTEN-FREE**
✓ **ONE POT**
✓ **VEGAN**

2 pounds sweet potatoes, peeled and cut in half

¾ to 1 cup orange juice

1½ tablespoons ginger paste

2 teaspoons ground cinnamon

1 teaspoon vanilla extract

½ cup chopped pecans

1. Put the sweet potatoes in a pot and cover with water. Bring to a boil and cook for 30 to 35 minutes, or until soft. Drain water.

2. Add the orange juice, ginger paste, cinnamon, and vanilla. Using a hand mixer, beat the ingredients together until no longer chunky.

3. Stir in pecans and serve hot.

VARIATION TIP: Add chopped walnuts or nutmeg instead of the pecans and cinnamon for a change in flavor.

PER SERVING: Total Calories: 210; Total Fat: 7g; Saturated Fat: 1g; Cholesterol: 0mg; Sodium: 83mg; Potassium: 613mg; Total Carbohydrate: 36g; Fiber: 6g; Sugars: 9g; Protein: 4g

KALE STRAWBERRY SALAD

SERVES 8 **PREP TIME** 15 MINUTES

Kale is a nutritional powerhouse. This leafy green is often dismissed because of its rough texture, but if you massage it with olive oil, the leaves wilt and sweeten a bit. Kale is a good source of potassium to help lower blood pressure, and are only 25 calories per cup. This crisp spring salad also features strawberries, which are an excellent source of vitamin C to promote a strong immune system. You could also add raspberries or blueberries for more variety and fiber. Adding grilled chicken, fish, or shrimp makes this salad a meal. Bon appétit!

✓ **30-MINUTE**

✓ **DIABETIC FRIENDLY**

✓ **GLUTEN-FREE**

✓ **ONE POT**

✓ **VEGETARIAN**

1 bunch curly kale, rinsed and dried

1 teaspoon olive oil

2 cups strawberries

¼ red onion, thinly cut into rings

⅔ cup chopped walnuts or pecans

¼ cup shredded Parmesan cheese

2 tablespoons corn oil

2 tablespoons balsamic vinegar

1 teaspoon Dijon mustard

1 teaspoon honey

1. Place kale and olive oil in a resealable plastic bag. Massage the kale and olive oil together until the kale is shiny; then remove from the bag and place in a medium bowl.

2. Cut the berries into small chunks and add to the bowl. Add the red onion, chopped nuts, and Parmesan cheese.

3. In a separate bowl, whisk together the corn oil, vinegar, mustard, and honey until well incorporated.

4. Drizzle dressing over the salad, and toss right before serving.

SUBSTITUTION TIP: Plumb out of balsamic vinegar? No problem. Red wine vinegar or apple cider vinegar will do just fine. You could also try feta or blue cheese instead of Parmesan.

PER SERVING: Total Calories: 169; Total Fat: 11g; Saturated Fat: 2g; Cholesterol: 3mg; Sodium: 77mg; Potassium: 514mg; Total Carbohydrate: 15g; Fiber: 3g; Sugars: 4g; Protein: 5g

SESAME GINGER BROCCOLI SLAW

SERVES 6 **PREP TIME** 5 MINUTES **COOK TIME** 15 MINUTES

The woody stalks of broccoli are often discarded in favor of florets—but don't toss them out! Combine them with shredded carrots and red cabbage to make broccoli slaw, a powerhouse salad packed with color and nutrients such as vitamin K and beta-carotene. Broccoli is low in purines and high in anti-inflammatory antioxidants, including vitamin C. It's also an excellent source of folate, potassium, and sulforaphane—a powerful phytochemical that reduces inflammation and helps prevent cancer. To make your life easier, you can find packaged broccoli slaw at any major grocery store.

✓ **30-MINUTE**
✓ **DIABETIC FRIENDLY**
✓ **GLUTEN-FREE**
✓ **KIDNEY FRIENDLY**
✓ **ONE POT**
✓ **VEGAN**

2 cups broccoli slaw

½ cup slivered almonds

¼ cup canola or corn oil

2 tablespoons lemon juice

1 teaspoon honey

1 teaspoon sesame oil

1 teaspoon low-sodium soy sauce

1 teaspoon ginger paste

1 garlic clove, minced

½ cup chopped cilantro

1. In a medium bowl, combine the broccoli slaw and almonds.

2. In a separate bowl, whisk together the canola oil, lemon juice, honey, sesame oil, soy sauce, ginger paste, and garlic.

3. Add the dressing to the broccoli slaw and toss. Mix in the chopped cilantro at the end, saving a few leaves for garnish. Slaw can be served alone or used in fish tacos.

SUBSTITUTION TIP: Agave nectar or maple syrup works great in place of honey.

PER SERVING: Total Calories: 150; Total Fat: 14g; Saturated Fat: 2g; Cholesterol: 0mg; Sodium: 41mg; Potassium: 176mg; Total Carbohydrate: 5g; Fiber: 2g; Sugars: 2g; Protein: 3g

SPINACH SALAD WITH POMEGRANATE AND PEARS

SERVES 4 **PREP TIME** 10 MINUTES

This seasonal salad is not only pretty but highly nutritious. Baby spinach provides beta-carotene, vitamin C, and potassium; pears and pomegranate seeds boost the fiber content. Crisp, crimson pomegranate seeds are a welcome change to traditional chewy dried cranberries. Maple syrup sweetens the apple cider vinegar dressing nicely, and blue cheese "pears" beautifully with fresh pears, spinach, and arugula.

✓ **30-MINUTE**
✓ **DIABETIC FRIENDLY**
✓ **GLUTEN-FREE**
✓ **ONE POT**
✓ **VEGETARIAN**

12 cups organic
 baby spinach

2 D'Anjou or comice pears

¼ cup chopped walnuts

¼ cup blue cheese crumbles

⅓ cup apple cider vinegar

⅓ cup canola oil

1 teaspoon Dijon mustard

2 teaspoons pure
 maple syrup

Seeds from 1 pomegranate

1. Wash and spin the greens in a salad spinner, or rinse thoroughly and pat dry; then place in a large salad bowl.

2. Cut the pears into wedges and place on top of the greens. Sprinkle walnuts and blue cheese over the salad and toss.

3. In a separate bowl, whisk together the vinegar, canola oil, mustard, and maple syrup. Drizzle over the salad and toss.

4. Garnish with pomegranate seeds and serve.

SUBSTITUTION TIP: You can use chopped pecans instead of walnuts.

PER SERVING: Total Calories: 331; Total Fat: 25g; Saturated Fat: 3g; Cholesterol: 9mg; Sodium: 188mg; Potassium: 673mg; Total Carbohydrate: 24g; Fiber: 6g; Sugars: 14g; Protein: 5g

CHILI GARLIC GREEN BEANS

SERVES 4 **PREP TIME** 10 MINUTES **COOK TIME** 10

Most Americans don't eat the recommended number of vegetable servings each day, but this recipe can help change that. Fresh or frozen green beans, which are low in calories but a good source of vitamin C, take on a whole new flavor with this chili garlic sauce. This is a great side dish to serve with Black Peppercorn Pork (page 96).

✓ **30-MINUTE**
✓ **DIABETIC FRIENDLY**
✓ **GLUTEN-FREE**
✓ **ONE POT**
✓ **VEGAN**

1 pound fresh green beans

1 teaspoon water

2 tablespoons low-sodium soy sauce

1 garlic clove, minced

1 teaspoon chili garlic sauce

2 teaspoons canola or vegetable oil

1. In a microwave-safe dish, combine the green beans with water and cover. Microwave the green beans for 3 to 4 minutes, or until the beans are bright green but slightly soft.

2. In a small bowl, whisk the soy sauce, garlic, and chili garlic sauce together and set aside.

3. Heat the canola oil in a medium skillet. Add the green beans and sauté for 3 to 4 minutes.

4. Pour the soy sauce mixture over the green beans, cover the skillet, and cook on low heat for another 2 minutes. Serve the beans hot.

VARIATION TIP: Minced ginger or ginger paste can be added to give the green beans for extra flavor.

PER SERVING: Total Calories: 62; Total Fat: 3g; Saturated Fat: 0g; Cholesterol: 0mg; Sodium: 307mg; Potassium: 256mg; Total Carbohydrate: 9g; Fiber: 4g; Sugars: 2g; Protein: 3g

TOMATO WATERMELON SALAD

SERVES 4   **PREP TIME** 10 MINUTES

I know, this sounds like a strange combination of produce. But trust me—you won't be sorry with this seasonal salad. Tomatoes and watermelon are both great sources of beta-carotene, vitamin C, potassium, and cancer-fighting lycopene. Putting them over a bed of romaine boosts the volume and fiber as well as adding beautiful color. Fresh basil adds a little twist.

✓ **30-MINUTE**
✓ **DIABETIC FRIENDLY**
✓ **GLUTEN-FREE**
✓ **ONE POT**
✓ **VEGAN**

5 cups seeded watermelon, cut into ¾-inch cubes

1½ pounds tomatoes, cut into ¾-inch cubes

3 teaspoons sugar

½ teaspoon salt

1 small red onion, quartered and thinly sliced

½ cup red wine vinegar

¼ cup extra-virgin olive oil

Cracked black pepper

½ cup fresh basil leaves, chopped

Romaine lettuce leaves (optional)

1. In a large bowl, combine watermelon and tomatoes. Sprinkle with sugar and salt, tossing to coat. Let stand 15 minutes.

2. Add the onion, vinegar, and oil, and toss. Cover and chill 2 hours.

3. Sprinkle with cracked black pepper and basil. Serve chilled with lettuce leaves (if using).

VARIATION TIP: Substitute fresh mint leaves for basil to change things up.

PER SERVING: Total Calories: 221; Total Fat: 13g; Saturated Fat: 2g; Cholesterol: 0mg; Sodium: 304mg; Potassium: 671mg; Total Carbohydrate: 26g; Fiber: 3g; Sugars: 20g; Protein: 3g

ARUGULA AND SPINACH SALAD IN CITRUS DRESSING

SERVES 4 **PREP TIME** 5 MINUTES

This seasonal salad will become a favorite among family and friends. Raspberries offer beautiful color as well as antioxidants and fiber, and they complement the flavors of the arugula, baby spinach, and fresh lime vinaigrette. Blue cheese and pecans further enhance the flavor, but you could use other cheeses (like feta) and any nuts or seeds you like. Grilled chicken or fish could be added to make this salad a complete meal.

✓ **30-MINUTE**
✓ **DIABETIC FRIENDLY**
✓ **GLUTEN-FREE**
✓ **ONE POT**
✓ **VEGETARIAN**

3 cups baby spinach leaves or local microgreens

3 cups arugula

2 pints fresh raspberries

¼ cup chopped pecans

¼ cup blue cheese crumbles (optional)

⅓ cup fresh lime juice

⅓ cup canola oil

1 teaspoon honey

1. Wash and spin the spinach and arugula in a salad spinner, or rinse and pat dry; then place in a large salad bowl.

2. Clean and dry the raspberries and add to the greens. Add the pecans and blue cheese (if using).

3. In a separate bowl, whisk together the lime juice, canola oil, and honey. Pour over salad and toss before serving.

VARIATION TIP: Blueberries and lemon juice can be substituted for raspberries and lime juice to change up the salad's flavor.

PER SERVING: Total Calories: 310; Total Fat: 24g; Saturated Fat: 2g; Cholesterol: 0mg; Sodium: 24mg; Potassium: 483mg; Total Carbohydrate: 25g; Fiber: 12g; Sugars: 10g; Protein: 4g

FIESTA RICE

SERVES 6 **PREP TIME** 10 MINUTES **COOK TIME** 45 MINUTES

No more bland rice! This colorful dish can be enjoyed any time of year. Fresh veggies add color, flavor, and phytochemicals, while cumin and garlic kick up the spice. I love serving it with Coconut Spice Chicken in Pita (page 86) or Dillicious Fish with Roasted Broccoli (page 66).

✓ **GLUTEN-FREE**

✓ **ONE POT**

2 tablespoons olive oil

1 (10-ounce) package frozen corn

1 tablespoon butter

1 cup chopped green onions (white and green parts)

1½ cups brown rice

2 garlic cloves, minced

1 teaspoon ground cumin

2 cups low-sodium chicken broth

1 teaspoon salt

⅛ teaspoon freshly ground black pepper

½ cup chopped fresh cilantro

1 tablespoon fresh lime juice

1. Heat the oil in a medium pot over medium heat. Add the corn to the pan and cook for 8 to 10 minutes, stirring occasionally, or until corn starts to brown. Remove from the pot and set aside.

2. In the same pot, melt the butter. Add the onions and sauté until soft. Add the rice, garlic, and cumin, and cook for 1 minute.

3. Add the chicken broth, salt, and pepper. Cover and bring to a boil. Cook for 5 minutes, and then reduce heat to low and simmer for 40 to 45 minutes, stirring occasionally.

4. When the rice has soaked up all the broth, add the corn back to the pot along with the cilantro and lime juice. Serve immediately.

COOKING TIP: This dish can be made in an electric pressure cooker if you've got one. Set the pot to "Sauté." With the lid open, add the corn and oil and stir for 5 to 6 minutes, or until corn is browned. Add the butter, onions, rice, cumin, and garlic and cook for 3 to 4 minutes, or until onions are soft. Add 1½ cups of chicken broth, and the salt and pepper, and close the lid to steam. Set the cooker on "Rice" and allow to cook until the cycle finishes (10 to 15 minutes). Release the pressure and serve the rice hot. Garnish the rice with cilantro and a squeeze of lime juice.

PER SERVING: Total Calories: 275; Total Fat: 8g; Saturated Fat: 2g; Cholesterol: 5mg; Sodium: 453mg; Potassium: 302mg; Total Carbohydrate: 48g; Fiber: 4g; Sugars: 2g; Protein: 6g

CURRY ROASTED CAULIFLOWER

SERVES 6 **PREP TIME** 5 MINUTES **COOK TIME** 30 MINUTES

Don't lump cauliflower in the group of "white foods" to avoid because it's not the same as white bread, white rice, and white sugar, which tend to raise blood sugar. As a member of the anti-inflammatory cabbage family, cauliflower is a nutritional boss. But don't just rice it! Roasting it with onions and curry powder turns it into a delightfully flavorful side dish.

✓ **DIABETIC FRIENDLY**
✓ **GLUTEN-FREE**
✓ **ONE POT**
✓ **VEGETARIAN**

4 garlic cloves, sliced

2 tablespoons lemon juice

⅓ cup olive oil

1½ teaspoons yellow curry powder

1 teaspoon ground cumin

½ teaspoon salt

¼ teaspoon freshly ground pepper

1 large cauliflower head, cut into large florets

½ white or yellow onion, sliced thick

1. Position the oven rack 8 inches from the top. Preheat the oven to 425°F. Line a large baking sheet with parchment paper.

2. Whisk the garlic, lemon juice, olive oil, curry powder, cumin, salt, and pepper together in a large bowl. Add the cauliflower and onion and mix to coat.

3. Arrange cauliflower and onion on the baking sheet in a single layer.

4. Roast for 10 to 15 minutes; then flip cauliflower and onion slices and roast another 10 to 15 minutes, or until browned. Serve immediately.

SUBSTITUTION TIP: For a sweet and savory flavor, substitute cinnamon for cumin.

PER SERVING: Total Calories: 142; Total Fat: 12g; Saturated Fat: 2g; Cholesterol: 0mg; Sodium: 238mg; Potassium: 467mg; Total Carbohydrate: 10g; Fiber: 4g; Sugars: 4g; Protein: 3g

SPICY PUMPKIN COCONUT SOUP

SERVES 6   **PREP TIME** 15 MINUTES   **COOK TIME** 40 MINUTES

Pumpkin is more versatile than you think. This recipe takes everyone's fall favorite and pairs it with cinnamon, nutmeg, and coconut milk to make a creamy soup. Pumpkin is an excellent source of the antioxidants beta-carotene and vitamin C as well as potassium. Top this soup with crunchy pumpkin seeds or chopped pecans for extra crunch.

✓ **DIABETIC FRIENDLY**
✓ **GLUTEN-FREE**
✓ **ONE POT**
✓ **VEGETARIAN**

3 tablespoons canola oil

1 large yellow
  onion, chopped

4 garlic cloves, minced

½ teaspoon sea salt

2 (15-ounce) cans
  pumpkin purée

½ teaspoon
  ground cinnamon

½ teaspoon ground nutmeg

¼ teaspoon ground cloves

4 cups vegetable broth

¼ cup green pumpkin
  seeds (pepitas)

½ cup light coconut milk

2 tablespoons honey

Fresh cilantro, for garnish
  (optional)

Freshly ground pepper, for
  topping (optional)

1. Heat the canola oil in a large pot or Dutch oven. Add the onion, garlic, and sea salt, and cook until the onion is soft and translucent.

2. Stir in pumpkin, cinnamon, nutmeg, and cloves. Add vegetable broth and bring the mixture to a boil for 5 minutes. Reduce the heat and simmer on low for about 15 minutes.

3. While soup is cooking, toast the pumpkin seeds in a dry skillet, tossing regularly, about 5 minutes. Set aside when done.

4. Add coconut milk and honey to the pumpkin soup. Cook until heated through. Top with fresh cilantro and pepper, if desired.

VARIATION TIP: Cumin and curry can replace the cinnamon and nutmeg to make a more savory soup.

PER SERVING: Total Calories: 245; Total Fat: 15g; Saturated Fat: 6g; Cholesterol: 0mg; Sodium: 678mg; Potassium: 529mg; Total Carbohydrate: 23g; Fiber: 5g; Sugars: 13g; Protein: 7g

ROASTED BRUSSELS SPROUTS WITH HORSERADISH MUSTARD

SERVES 4 **PREP TIME** 15 MINUTES **COOK TIME** 15 MINUTES

Don't settle for boring Brussels sprouts! Horseradish mustard gives these baby cabbages a tangy flavor without extra fat, sugar, or salt. Brussels sprouts are chock-full of anti-inflammatory compounds that make them gout-friendly. This dish is so easy to make, you can enjoy it regularly.

✓ **30-MINUTE**
✓ **DIABETIC FRIENDLY**
✓ **GLUTEN-FREE**
✓ **ONE POT**
✓ **VEGETARIAN**

½ cup water

2 tablespoons olive oil

1 tablespoon butter

1 pound fresh Brussels sprouts, trimmed of yellow leaves

2 tablespoons horseradish mustard

½ teaspoon salt

¼ teaspoon freshly ground black pepper

1. In a large skillet or Dutch oven, bring water, olive oil, and butter to a boil and cook for 3 minutes.

2. Add the Brussels sprouts, cover, and steam over medium heat until bright green and soft, 5 to 10 minutes.

3. Remove the lid and sauté for 1 to 2 minutes, or until the liquid evaporates.

4. Add the mustard, salt, and pepper to the Brussels sprouts, and toss before serving.

VARIATION TIP: If you'd like a milder flavor than horseradish, you can use honey mustard or Dijon mustard instead.

PER SERVING: Total Calories: 142; Total Fat: 10g; Saturated Fat: 3g; Cholesterol: 8mg; Sodium: 460mg; Potassium: 443mg; Total Carbohydrate: 10g; Fiber: 4g; Sugars: 3g; Protein: 4g

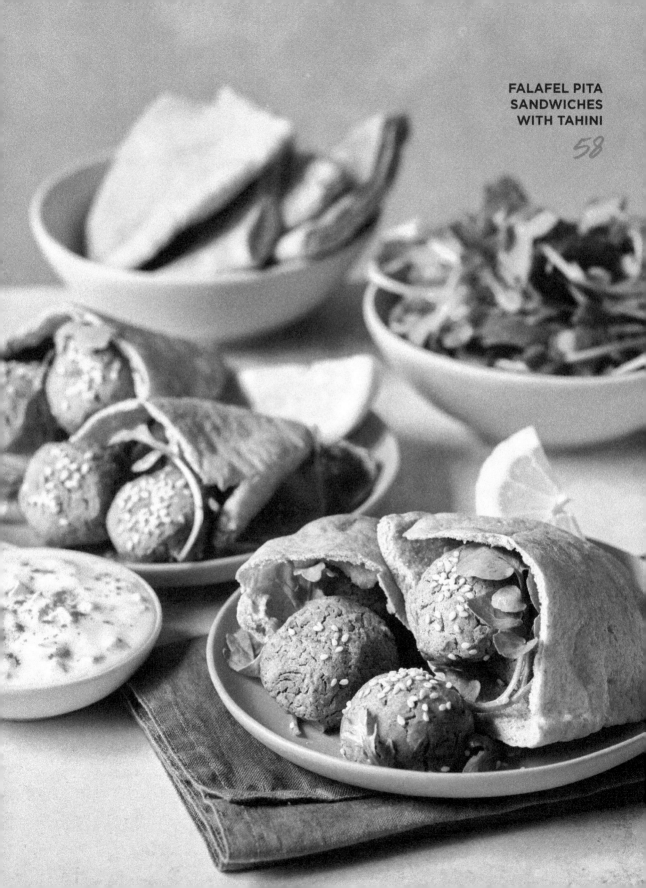

Vegetarian Entrées

Here is a whole chapter devoted to meatless meals! All the dishes are plant-based and include a variety of full-flavored whole grains, beans, and other protein sources. You can try recipes like Lentil Quinoa Salad with Dried Cherries and Pecans (page 54), Falafel Pita Sandwiches with Tahini (page 58), and Chipotle Black Bean and Sweet Potato Bowl with Farro (page 55). Meatless Mondays just got a lot more interesting.

SAVORY RED LENTIL STEW

SERVES 6   **PREP TIME** 10 MINUTES   **COOK TIME** 30 MINUTES

Did you know that spices such as curry powder have anti-inflammatory effects? This simple dish is inspired by *masoor dal*, a lentil curry that is a staple of Indian cuisine and perfect for a cool fall day. It is an excellent source of dietary fiber, potassium, protein, fiber, and iron—a nutrient that is difficult to obtain in vegetarian diets. Serve it over rice or with a loaf of warm, crusty bread or naan (traditional Indian bread). You won't be disappointed!

✓ **GLUTEN-FREE**

✓ **VEGAN**

2 tablespoons olive oil

1 yellow or white
 onion, chopped

2 garlic cloves, minced

2 teaspoons ginger paste

1 tablespoon ground cumin

1 tablespoon yellow
 curry powder

1 teaspoon salt

1 (15-ounce) can
 diced tomatoes

1 cup red lentils, rinsed

4 cups water, divided

1 cup basmati rice

2 tablespoons
 cilantro, chopped, for
 garnish (optional)

1. Heat the olive oil in a large pan. Add the onion and sauté for 5 minutes.

2. Add the garlic, ginger paste, cumin, curry powder, and salt, and stir to combine. Add the diced tomatoes and cook until the tomatoes are soft.

3. Add the lentils and 2 cups of water to the mixture and cook for roughly 30 minutes, or until lentils are soft.

4. While the lentils are cooking, combine the remaining 2 cups of water and rice in a separate pot. Bring to a boil and cook for 20 to 30 minutes, or until rice is soft.

5. Serve the lentils over basmati rice, garnished with cilantro (if using).

SUBSTITUTION TIP: Canola or corn oil can be used instead of olive oil.

PER SERVING: Total Calories: 296; Total Fat: 6g; Saturated Fat: 1g; Cholesterol: 0mg; Sodium: 398mg; Potassium: 582mg; Total Carbohydrate: 50g; Fiber: 12g; Sugars: 3g; Protein: 12g

BLACK BEAN CHILI

SERVES 4 **PREP TIME** 5 MINUTES **COOK TIME** 20 MINUTES

This simple recipe is not only super quick but very healthy. Beans provide a hefty dose of belly-filling fiber as well as protein, potassium, folate, and magnesium. Adding tomatoes or bell peppers (which are high in vitamin C) increases the iron absorption from the beans. Leftover chili is great served over rice or in tortillas for burritos.

✓ **30-MINUTE**

✓ **GLUTEN-FREE**

✓ **ONE POT**

✓ **VEGAN**

1 (10-ounce) can diced tomatoes with green chilies

½ onion, chopped

1 garlic clove, minced

2 teaspoons ground cumin

1 teaspoon dried oregano

1 teaspoon chili powder

2 (15-ounce) cans black beans, drained and rinsed

½ to 1 teaspoon salt

2% milk shredded cheese, for serving

1. In a medium saucepan, combine the tomatoes, onion, garlic, cumin, oregano, and chili powder. Simmer until the vegetables are soft.

2. Add the beans and cook for another 10 to 15 minutes, or until the beans are soft. Stir in salt to taste. Serve with shredded cheese.

SUBSTITUTION TIP: You can use kidney beans or pinto beans instead of black beans.

COOKING TIP: Draining and rinsing the beans reduces the sodium content by 30 percent.

PER SERVING: Total Calories: 326; Total Fat: 7g; Saturated Fat: 4g; Cholesterol: 20mg; Sodium: 603mg; Potassium: 931mg; Total Carbohydrate: 45g; Fiber: 16g; Sugars: 7g; Protein: 23g

PIZZA SOUP

SERVES 8   **PREP TIME** 10 MINUTES   **COOK TIME** 20 MINUTES

This pizza soup has all the delicious elements of pizza, minus the crust! This recipe is a perfect representation of the Mediterranean diet—gout-friendly and vegetarian to boot. The Mediterranean diet is a plant-based eating style based on the dietary habits of populations living near the Mediterranean (Greece, Italy, France, Spain, etc.). It emphasizes fruits, vegetables, beans, whole grains, lean meats, and low-fat dairy products and has been shown to reduce the risk of heart disease and diabetes. This pizza soup is not only high in fiber, it's also a great source of protein, potassium, vitamin C, and cancer-fighting phytochemicals. Top with shredded Parmesan or Asiago cheese and serve with a rustic, crusty bread and you'll feel like you're in old Italy.

✓ **30-MINUTE**

✓ **DIABETIC FRIENDLY**

✓ **GLUTEN-FREE**

✓ **ONE POT**

✓ **VEGETARIAN**

2 tablespoons olive oil

½ onion, chopped

1 garlic clove, minced

1 tablespoon dried oregano

1 tablespoon dried basil

1 tablespoon dried rosemary

6 cups chicken or
   vegetable broth

1 (15-ounce) can diced
   tomatoes with the liquid

1 box chopped frozen
   spinach, thawed

2 (15-ounce) cans white
   beans, drained and rinsed

Shredded Parmesan or
   Asiago cheese, for serving

Bread, for serving (optional)

1. Heat the olive oil in a large pot. Add the onion, garlic, oregano, basil, and rosemary, and sauté until the onion is translucent.

2. Add the broth, tomatoes, spinach, and white beans, and continue to simmer on medium heat until soup thickens, about 20 minutes.

3. Serve with shredded Parmesan or Asiago cheese and your favorite bread (if using).

VARIATION TIP: Chopped fresh fennel or thyme can be added at the end for a different flavor.

COOKING TIP: Cooking the onions, garlic, and spices in a little olive oil makes them more aromatic, but you can also leave the oil out and cook them in the diced tomatoes.

PER SERVING: Total Calories: 244; Total Fat: 8g; Saturated Fat: 3g; Cholesterol: 13mg; Sodium: 474mg; Potassium: 635mg; Total Carbohydrate: 32g; Fiber: 11g; Sugars: 3g; Protein: 14g

WHITE BEAN AND KALE SOUP

SERVES 8   **PREP TIME** 10 MINUTES   **COOK TIME** 25 MINUTES

This soup may sound bland at first glance, but it will surprise you with its full body and flavor. The combination of kale, carrots, and beans provides a double dose of fiber, potassium, and disease-fighting beta-carotene. You can also use fresh or frozen spinach in place of kale.

✓ **DIABETIC FRIENDLY**
✓ **GLUTEN-FREE**
✓ **ONE POT**
✓ **VEGAN**

1 small white or yellow onion, chopped

2 tablespoons canola oil

2 garlic cloves, minced

2 large carrots, diced

2 celery stalks, chopped

1 large bunch curly kale, chopped

1 tablespoon Italian seasoning

4 cups low-sodium vegetable broth

2 (15-ounce) cans great northern or navy beans, drained and rinsed

Shredded Parmesan cheese, for serving (optional)

1. In a large soup pot, sauté the onion in canola oil until translucent.

2. Add the garlic, followed by the carrots, celery, kale, and Italian seasoning. Continue to cook on low heat until the vegetables are soft and well seasoned.

3. Add the vegetable broth and the beans, and simmer on low for another 20 minutes.

4. Soup can be served with a teaspoon of shredded Parmesan cheese (if using).

TRIGGER TIP: If a flare-up has affected your hands, you can use frozen mirepoix (a mixture of finely chopped onions, carrots, and celery) and a box of frozen spinach instead of chopping all the vegetables.

PER SERVING: Total Calories: 177; Total Fat: 5g; Saturated Fat: 0g; Cholesterol: 1mg; Sodium: 235mg; Potassium: 597mg; Total Carbohydrate: 27g; Fiber: 9g; Sugars: 2g; Protein: 9g

LENTIL QUINOA SALAD WITH DRIED CHERRIES AND PECANS

SERVES 6   **PREP TIME** 5 MINUTES, PLUS 1 HOUR TO CHILL   **COOK TIME** 45 MINUTES

This beautiful salad is not only colorful and delicious, it's a good source of fiber and antioxidants from the lentils, quinoa (a hearty ancient grain that's high in protein and fiber), and dried cherries. You can assemble it ahead of time, which makes it ideal for potlucks, picnics, and barbecues.

✓ **GLUTEN-FREE**

✓ **VEGETARIAN**

1 cup dry red lentils

4 cups water, divided

1 cup quinoa

3 tablespoons lemon juice

3 tablespoons canola oil

1 tablespoon apple cider vinegar

1 teaspoon honey

½ cup pecans, chopped

½ cup dried cherries

½ cup feta cheese crumbles

1 green onion (green and white parts), chopped

1. In a medium pot, add the lentils to 2 cups of water and bring to a boil. Cook for 3 minutes; then reduce heat to low and simmer until the lentils are soft, about 30 minutes. Drain off extra water and place in a large bowl to cool.

2. While the lentils are cooking, bring the quinoa and the remaining 2 cups of water to a boil. Cook for 3 minutes; then cover the pot, reduce heat, and continue to simmer for about 15 minutes, or until the water has been absorbed. Allow quinoa to cool, and then add it to the cooled lentils.

3. Pour lemon juice into a microwave-safe bowl, and micro-wave for 30 seconds. Add the canola oil, vinegar, and honey, and whisk to make a dressing.

4. Pour the dressing over the lentils and quinoa. Add the pecans, cherries, feta cheese, and green onions, and toss the salad to coat. Refrigerate for at least 1 hour before serving.

VARIATION TIP: Balsamic vinegar and Dijon mustard can be used in place of apple cider vinegar, canola oil, and honey to make a richer dressing.

PER SERVING: Total Calories: 394; Total Fat: 18g; Saturated Fat: 3g; Cholesterol: 7mg; Sodium: 117mg; Potassium: 521mg; Total Carbohydrate: 46g; Fiber: 13g; Sugars: 7g; Protein: 15g

CHIPOTLE BLACK BEAN AND SWEET POTATO BOWL WITH FARRO

SERVES 4 **PREP TIME** 10 MINUTES **COOK TIME** 30 MINUTES

This dish is a bit more labor-intensive than some of the others in this chapter but worth every bite. Chipotle chili powder and fresh lime juice combine to create a deliciously bold dish using sweet potatoes, fresh spinach, avocado, and farro. This bowl is a good source of potassium, which helps lower blood pressure.

✓ VEGETARIAN

1 pound sweet potatoes, peeled and diced

2½ tablespoons canola oil, divided

1 teaspoon chipotle chili powder, divided

1 teaspoon salt, divided

½ teaspoon freshly ground black pepper, divided

1 large red or yellow bell pepper, quartered

3 cups water

1 cup dry farro

2 tablespoons fresh lime juice

1 teaspoon lime zest

1 tablespoon fresh cilantro, chopped

4 cups baby spinach

1 avocado, cut into 1-inch chunks

¼ cup feta cheese crumbles

1. Preheat oven to 400°F. Line a large baking sheet with aluminum foil.

2. In a large mixing bowl, combine the sweet potatoes, ½ tablespoon of canola oil, ½ teaspoon of chipotle chili powder, ⅛ teaspoon of salt, and ¼ teaspoon of pepper.

3. Place the seasoned sweet potatoes on one side of the pan and the bell peppers on the other side of the pan. Brush the peppers with ½ tablespoon of canola oil. Bake the potatoes and peppers for about 30 minutes, or until the potatoes are soft and peppers are slightly charred.

4. While the vegetables are baking, place the water and farro in a medium saucepan. Bring to a boil and cook for 5 minutes. Reduce the heat, cover the pot, and simmer for 20 minutes, or until farro is soft. Drain the farro and set aside.

5. Whisk together the remaining 1½ tablespoons of canola oil, ½ teaspoon of chipotle chili powder, ½ teaspoon of salt, ¼ teaspoon of pepper, lime juice, lime zest, and cilantro.

6. Divide farro among 4 bowls. Top with sweet potatoes, spinach, and avocado chunks. Drizzle lime dressing over the bowls and top with feta cheese.

SUBSTITUTION TIP: You can use quinoa or brown rice instead of farro to make the recipe gluten-free.

PER SERVING: Total Calories: 421; Total Fat: 19g; Saturated Fat: 3g; Cholesterol: 8mg; Sodium: 195mg; Potassium: 845mg; Total Carbohydrate: 55g; Fiber: 12g; Sugars: 7g; Protein: 10g

PASTA FAGIOLI

SERVES 6   **PREP TIME** 8 MINUTES   **COOK TIME** 20 MINUTES

This classic Italian recipe is the perfect comfort food for a cold day. Curl up with a bowl of this and all your troubles will melt away. Not only is the tomato-based sauce hearty, but it's a great source of antioxidants, including vitamin C and lycopene. This dish is also a great source of fiber and potassium, thanks to the whole-grain pasta, beans, and veggies.

✓ **30-MINUTE**

✓ **VEGAN**

2 tablespoons olive oil

1 carrot, diced

1 celery stalk, diced

¼ cup chopped onion

1 tablespoon paprika

1 garlic clove, minced

2 (15-ounce) cans tomato sauce

1 (14-ounce) can vegetable broth

1 (15-ounce) can cannellini beans, drained and rinsed

1 tablespoon dried basil

1½ cups whole-wheat ditalini or elbow pasta

1 cup shredded Parmesan cheese (optional)

1. Heat the olive oil in a medium saucepan. Add the carrot, celery, and onion, and sauté until the onion is soft. Add the paprika and garlic and sauté another 3 minutes.

2. Add the tomato sauce, vegetable broth, cannellini beans, and basil to the vegetables and simmer on low heat for 15 minutes.

3. While the beans are cooking, use a separate pot to cook the pasta for about 8 minutes, or until al dente. Drain the pasta and add it to the soup mixture. Mix well and serve with shredded Parmesan cheese (if using).

SUBSTITUTION TIP: You can use great northern or navy beans if you don't have cannellini beans on hand.

PER SERVING: Total Calories: 237; Total Fat: 6g; Saturated Fat: 1g; Cholesterol: 0mg; Sodium: 832mg; Potassium: 681mg; Total Carbohydrate: 41g; Fiber: 9g; Sugars: 8g; Protein: 10g

SAUCY JAMAICAN KIDNEY BEANS WITH RICE

SERVES 4 **PREP TIME** 5 MINUTES **COOK TIME** 30 MINUTES

This delicious dish features traditional Jamaican flavors, including allspice and garlic. The inspiration for this recipe came when I attended a potluck with a Caribbean friend, who identified which flavors stood out most to him. Using light coconut milk reduces the saturated fat content of the meal. Kidney beans and brown rice provide a good dose of dietary fiber and make a complete protein.

✓ **GLUTEN-FREE**
✓ **ONE POT**
✓ **VEGAN**

1 (14-ounce) can light coconut milk

¼ cup water

1 tablespoon dried thyme

1 garlic clove, chopped

½ teaspoon allspice

½ teaspoon salt

¼ teaspoon cayenne pepper

1 cup brown rice

1 (15-ounce) can dark red kidney beans

1. In a large pot over medium heat, combine the coconut milk, water, thyme, garlic, allspice, salt, and cayenne pepper. Simmer for 5 minutes.

2. Add the brown rice and cook for 20 minutes, or until rice is soft.

3. Stir in the kidney beans, cover the pot, and cook for 5 minutes to warm through prior to serving.

VARIATION TIP: For a sweeter taste, add minced ginger and cinnamon.

PER SERVING: Total Calories: 310; Total Fat: 7g; Saturated Fat: 5g; Cholesterol: 0mg; Sodium: 249mg; Potassium: 436mg; Total Carbohydrate: 54g; Fiber: 6g; Sugars: 0g; Protein: 11g

FALAFEL PITA SANDWICHES WITH TAHINI

SERVES 4 **PREP TIME** 20 MINUTES, PLUS 55 MINUTES TO CHILL **COOK TIME** 10 MINUTES

Falafel is a flavorful Mediterranean dish of mashed chickpeas, spices, and fresh herbs shaped into balls or patties and fried. The chickpeas are an excellent source of fiber, while the onions, garlic, parsley, and cilantro provide the antioxidants. Falafel can be served alone as an appetizer, but wrapping the patties in a pita to create a sandwich makes for a satisfying meal.

✓ **VEGETARIAN**

2 large onions, chopped

6 garlic cloves

1 (15-ounce) can chickpeas, drained

1 cup loosely packed fresh parsley leaves

1 cup loosely packed fresh cilantro leaves

1 teaspoon salt, divided

2 teaspoons ground cumin

2 teaspoons baking powder

Up to ½ cup white flour

1¼ cups plain low-fat Greek yogurt

¼ cup tahini

2 tablespoons lemon juice

Salt

Freshly ground black pepper

¼ cup corn or canola oil

Whole-wheat pita bread (4 pitas, cut in half)

Sesame seeds, for topping (optional)

Spring greens, for serving (optional)

1. Pulse the onion and garlic in a food processor until finely minced. Remove the mixture and place in a strainer, pressing down gently to get rid of as much liquid as possible; then set aside.

2. Combine the chickpeas, parsley, cilantro, ½ teaspoon of salt, and cumin in the food processor and pulse until they are roughly blended.

3. Put the onion and garlic mixture back into the food processor, and add the baking powder and a small amount of flour. Pulse the processor until the mixture forms a small ball, adding a little flour at a time as needed. The mixture should not be sticky. More flour can be added if it is too wet.

4. Move the falafel mixture to a small bowl and cover it with plastic wrap. Refrigerate for 1 hour.

5. While the falafel is chilling, prepare the tahini sauce. Whisk together the yogurt, tahini, and lemon juice. Season it with salt and pepper, and then put it in the refrigerator.

6. After the falafel mixture has chilled, form the mixture into balls using a small ice cream scoop or spoon, using about 3 tablespoons of mixture per ball. Flatten them into a patty shape. If the mixture is wet or sticky, more flour may be added.

7. In a large skillet, heat the corn oil. Preheat the oil for 3 minutes, and then add the falafel one at a time. Cook for 3 minutes per side, until browned and fully cooked.

8. Transfer the cooked falafel to a cooling rack or sheet pan lined with a paper towel.

9. Cut the pitas in half and place 3 or 4 falafel inside. Top the falafels with sesame seeds and stuff the pitas with spring greens, if desired. Serve with a side of tahini sauce.

SUBSTITUTION TIP: If you do not have tahini, you can use peanut butter instead.

PER SERVING: Total Calories: 639; Total Fat: 26g; Saturated Fat: 5g; Cholesterol: 5mg; Sodium: 1007mg; Potassium: 1158mg; Total Carbohydrate: 84g; Fiber: 14g; Sugars: 14g; Protein: 24g

VEGETARIAN BAKED ZITI

SERVES 8   **PREP TIME** 15 MINUTES   **COOK TIME** 45 MINUTES

You won't even miss the meat in this delicious Italian favorite. It takes a little longer, but it's totally worth the extra time. Using part-skim ricotta cheese cuts the fat and calories while providing a great source of calcium and protein. Tomato sauce brings a mighty dose of vitamin C, cancer-fighting lycopene, and potassium (which helps reduce blood pressure). All this to say, it's a delicious classic that's healthy too!

✓ **VEGETARIAN**

½ (8-ounce) box ziti or penne noodles

2 (8-ounce) cans tomato sauce

1 (4-ounce) can tomato paste

1 teaspoon prepared basil pesto

1 garlic clove, minced

1 teaspoon dried oregano

1 teaspoon dried rosemary

½ teaspoon salt

1 egg

1 (15-ounce) container part-skim ricotta cheese

½ cup shredded mozzarella cheese

1. Preheat the oven to 375°F.

2. In a medium pot, cook the ziti in boiling water for 8 minutes, or until al dente. Drain and set aside.

3. In another pot, combine the tomato sauce, tomato paste, pesto, garlic, oregano, rosemary, and salt. Stir together and simmer for about 10 minutes.

4. In a medium mixing bowl, combine the egg with the ricotta cheese.

5. Spread ½ cup of the sauce over the bottom of a 10-inch casserole dish. Cover the sauce with 1 cup of cooked ziti and then ½ cup of the ricotta mixture. Continue layering the sauce, noodles, and ricotta, ending with the remainder of the sauce on top.

6. Sprinkle mozzarella cheese over the top of the casserole and cover with aluminum foil or a lid.

7. Bake for 25 minutes, or until the cheese is bubbly. Let the dish rest for 5 minutes before serving.

SUBSTITUTION TIP: Use whole-wheat noodles to boost the fiber content.

PER SERVING: Total Calories: 233; Total Fat: 7g; Saturated Fat: 4g; Cholesterol: 41mg; Sodium: 583mg; Potassium: 411mg; Total Carbohydrate: 30g; Fiber: 2g; Sugars: 4g; Protein: 14g

CURRIED CHICKPEAS AND BASMATI RICE

SERVES 4 **PREP TIME** 5 MINUTES **COOK TIME** 25 MINUTES

If you're in a spicy mood, this is just the ticket! This recipe packs a flavorful punch with curry powder and garlic, not to mention sriracha. This dish features chickpeas (aka garbanzo beans), a great plant-based protein that's high in fiber and folate. Serve over rice—or add 4 cups of extra vegetable broth and make this dish into soup instead.

✓ **30-MINUTE**
✓ **GLUTEN-FREE**
✓ **VEGAN**

1 cup basmati rice

2 cups water

2 tablespoons canola oil

1 large onion, chopped

2 garlic cloves, minced

2 teaspoons curry powder

2 (15-ounce) cans chickpeas, drained and rinsed

1 (13.5-ounce) can reduced-fat coconut milk

1 cup vegetable broth

1 tablespoon honey

1 tablespoon sriracha sauce

Cilantro, chopped, for serving (optional)

1. In a pot, combine the basmati rice and bring to a boil. Cook for 3 minutes; then reduce heat and simmer for 12 to 15 minutes, or until the rice is cooked.

2. While the rice is cooking, heat the canola oil in a skillet over medium heat. Add the onion and sauté until caramelized, about 10 minutes.

3. Stir in the garlic and curry powder and cook for 1 minute. Add the chickpeas, coconut milk, vegetable broth, honey, and sriracha, and simmer for another 10 minutes. Serve over basmati rice with cilantro (if using).

VARIATION TIP: Cumin and cinnamon can be substituted for the curry powder for a different flavor.

PER SERVING: Total Calories: 530; Total Fat: 16g; Saturated Fat: 5g; Cholesterol: 0mg; Sodium: 227mg; Potassium: 542mg; Total Carbohydrate: 83g; Fiber: 11g; Sugars: 12g; Protein: 17g

VEGETARIAN ENCHILADAS

SERVES 6 **PREP TIME** 20 MINUTES **COOK TIME** 60 MINUTES

This recipe may look like it takes a lot of effort, but once you've finished your prep work on the stove, all you have to do is sit back and watch while dinner magically transforms in the oven. For spicier enchiladas, add chopped jalapeños to the filling or more cayenne pepper to the sauce. This meal comes with a hefty dose of protein, calcium, and fiber, and the rich tomato sauce and spinach give it an extra boost of vitamin C and potassium.

✓ **GLUTEN-FREE**

✓ **VEGETARIAN**

FOR THE SAUCE

2 tablespoons corn or olive oil

½ small onion, chopped

2 garlic cloves, minced

2 teaspoons chili powder

1 teaspoon ground cumin

Pinch cayenne pepper

1 (15-ounce) can tomato sauce

1 cup water

½ teaspoon salt

FOR THE FILLING

1 (10-ounce) package frozen spinach, thawed

1 (15-ounce) can black beans

1½ cups shredded sharp Cheddar cheese, divided

1½ cups shredded pepper Jack cheese, divided

½ cup light sour cream, divided

3 green onions, sliced (white and green parts), divided

12 corn tortillas

1 lime, juiced

1. Preheat the oven to 350°F.

2. To make the sauce, heat the corn oil in a large skillet. Add the onion and cook for about 5 minutes, or until soft. Add the garlic, chili powder, cumin, and cayenne pepper, and cook for 1 minute, stirring to coat the onions in seasoning. Add the tomato sauce, water, and salt, and continue to cook for 20 minutes, or until the sauce thickens.

3. For the filling, squeeze any excess liquid from the spinach. In a large bowl, place the spinach with the black beans.

4. Add ¾ cup of shredded Cheddar, ¾ cup of shredded pepper Jack cheese, ¼ cup of sour cream, and half of the green onions to the bean mixture.

5. In a 9-by-13-inch baking dish, spread ½ cup of sauce on the bottom of the pan. Place the corn tortillas flat on a clean work surface. Place ¼ cup of filling in each tortilla.

6. Roll the filled tortillas up and place them in rows in the baking dish.

7. Pour the remaining red tomato sauce over the enchiladas. Sprinkle the remaining ¾ cup of Cheddar cheese and ¾ cup of pepper Jack cheese on top.

8. Cover the enchilada pan loosely with aluminum foil and bake for 30 minutes. Uncover the enchiladas and bake for an additional 10 minutes.

9. In a small bowl, whisk together the remaining ¼ cup of sour cream and the lime juice. Drizzle over the enchiladas and serve.

SUBSTITUTION TIP: Out of black beans? Pinto beans or fat-free refried beans are a great substitute.

PER SERVING: Total Calories: 508; Total Fat: 25g; Saturated Fat: 15g; Cholesterol: 68mg; Sodium: 999mg; Potassium: 990mg; Total Carbohydrate: 50g; Fiber: 11g; Sugars: 6g; Protein: 26g

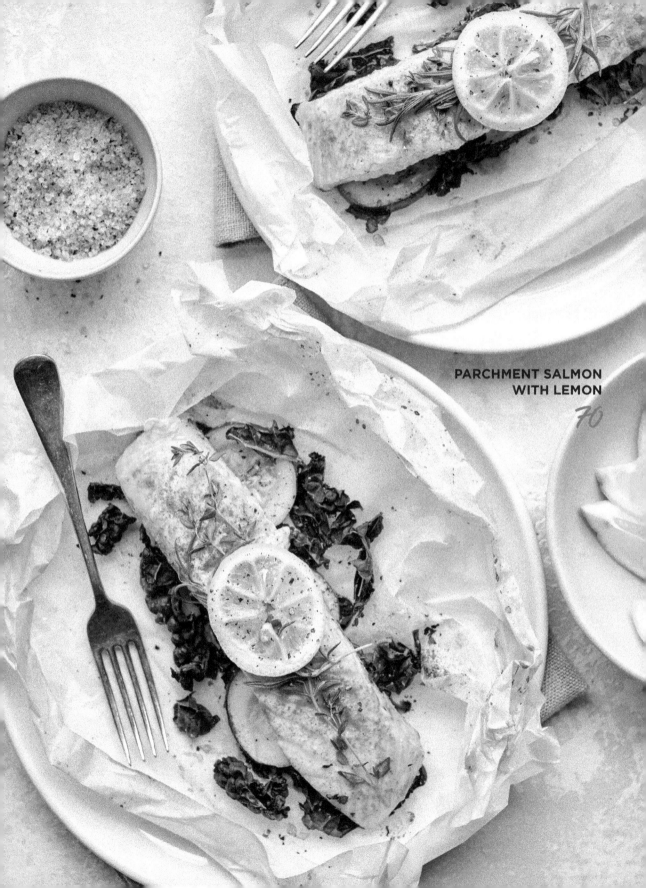

PARCHMENT SALMON
WITH LEMON

70

5

Fish and Seafood

Fish and seafood are becoming more popular, and with good reason. Eating fish twice a week may reduce the risk of heart disease. This chapter provides some tricks and tips for flavoring fish and seafood, with recipes like Broiled Tilapia with Herbed Mayonnaise (page 75), Tuna Steaks with Wasabi Sauce (page 72), and Honey Glazed Shrimp (page 68).

DILLICIOUS FISH WITH ROASTED BROCCOLI

SERVES 4   **PREP TIME** 5 MINUTES, PLUS 30 MINUTES TO MARINATE   **COOK TIME** 15 MINUTES

This recipe is super simple but really tasty. White fish such as tilapia is lower in purines than other types of fish, making it a gout-friendly food. If you're out of fresh lemons, use lemon juice from concentrate or 1 teaspoon lemon-pepper seasoning with 2 tablespoons of white vinegar. This fish can be baked, broiled, or grilled.

✓ **DIABETIC FRIENDLY**

✓ **GLUTEN-FREE**

2 tablespoons plus
  2 teaspoons olive
  oil, divided

2 tablespoons fresh
  lemon juice

1 teaspoon dried dill

½ teaspoon sea salt

4 tilapia fillets (about
  1 pound), fresh or frozen
  and thawed

1 broccoli head

Salt

Freshly ground black pepper

Lemon wedges, for
  serving (optional)

1. Preheat the oven to 400°F.

2. Whisk together 2 tablespoons of olive oil, the lemon juice, dill, and sea salt. Pour into a large resealable plastic bag. Add the fish and marinate for at least 30 minutes.

3. Cut broccoli into florets, leaving an inch of the stem on each one. Line a large baking sheet with parchment paper, and then spread the broccoli evenly on it.

4. Brush broccoli with the remaining 2 teaspoons of olive oil, and dust with salt and pepper. Roast the broccoli for 20 minutes.

5. Remove the broccoli from the oven and place the oven rack a few inches from the broiler. Line a broiling pan with aluminum foil and place the fish fillets on it. Broil for 4 to 6 minutes per side, or until the fish flakes.

6. Serve the fish with the roasted broccoli and lemon wedges (if using).

COOKING TIP: The fish can be prepared on the stove as well. Spray a large skillet with nonstick spray, and then heat over medium heat. Add the marinated fish fillets (two at a time) and cook for 5 to 6 minutes per side, or until the fish is flaky and completely cooked.

SUBSTITUTION TIP: Cauliflower or fresh carrots can be substituted for broccoli. Try a dusting of cumin on the vegetables for something different.

PER SERVING: Total Calories: 172; Total Fat: 5g; Saturated Fat: 1g; Cholesterol: 55mg; Sodium: 118mg; Potassium: 450mg; Total Carbohydrate: 9g; Fiber: 4g; Sugars: 3g; Protein: 25g

BROILED SALMON WITH BALSAMIC VINEGAR

SERVES 4 **PREP TIME** 5 MINUTES, PLUS 30 MINUTES TO MARINATE **COOK TIME** 15 MINUTES

It's no wonder that salmon is considered heart-healthy. Studies show that eating two servings of fatty fish per week can reduce your risk of heart disease and possibly dementia. Unlike certain varieties of fish, salmon is low in purines. It's an excellent source of omega-3 fatty acids, a type of fat found to reduce inflammation. On top of all the health benefits, this particular recipe pairs very nicely with colorful Fiesta Rice (page 43).

✓ **30-MINUTE**

✓ **DIABETIC FRIENDLY**

✓ **GLUTEN-FREE**

✓ **ONE POT**

6 tablespoons real maple syrup

2 tablespoons Dijon mustard

2 tablespoons balsamic vinegar

4 (3-ounce) salmon steaks or fillets

1. In a large mixing bowl or large resealable plastic bag, combine the maple syrup, mustard, and vinegar. Set aside 2 tablespoons of the marinade for basting.

2. Add the salmon to the bag and refrigerate. Marinate for at least 30 minutes but not longer than 12 hours.

3. Preheat the oven broiler when ready to cook the salmon, and line a broiling pan with aluminum foil. Broil the salmon fillets for 10 to 12 minutes, or until the fish is flaky and cooked through. Baste with the additional marinade and serve.

COOKING TIP: To save time and prepare a full meal, cook your Fiesta Rice while the fish is broiling.

PER SERVING: Total Calories: 271; Total Fat: 13g; Saturated Fat: 3g; Cholesterol: 46mg; Sodium: 134mg; Potassium: 83mg; Total Carbohydrate: 22g; Fiber: 1g; Sugars: 18g; Protein: 16g

HONEY GLAZED SHRIMP

SERVES 6   **PREP TIME** 5 MINUTES   **COOK TIME** 40 MINUTES

Shrimp adds variety to your diet, and it's also a quick-cooking protein. It's a safe sea-food to eat and won't exacerbate a gout flare-up. This recipe combines traditional seasonings with a touch of lemon, honey, and garlic. Instead of regular onions, I use shallots for their milder flavor, their pale purple color, and the hint of garlic they add to the dish. This shrimp pairs very well with Fiesta Rice (page 43) or Ginger Mashed Sweet Potatoes (page 36).

✓ **DIABETIC FRIENDLY**
✓ **GLUTEN-FREE**
✓ **KIDNEY FRIENDLY**
✓ **ONE POT**

2 pounds large shrimp, cleaned and drained

½ teaspoon salt

½ teaspoon freshly ground black pepper

1 teaspoon low-sodium Cajun or seafood seasoning

1 tablespoon olive oil

3 tablespoons lemon juice, divided

2 tablespoons honey

1 tablespoon butter

1 shallot, chopped

1 garlic clove, minced

1. Preheat an oven to 375°F. Lightly grease an 8-by-8-inch baking dish.

2. In a large bowl, season the shrimp with salt, pepper, and Cajun seasoning. Place the shrimp in the prepared baking dish and sprinkle with olive oil and 1 tablespoon of lemon juice.

3. Bake in preheated oven for 15 minutes, or until shrimp are hot and beginning to turn opaque.

4. In a small saucepan, combine the remaining 2 tablespoons of lemon juice with the honey, butter, shallot, and garlic, and simmer over medium heat. Cook and stir for 4 to 5 minutes, or until the sauce thickens and the shallot has softened and turned translucent.

5. Remove the shrimp from the oven and use tongs to flip each one over. Drizzle the hot lemon-honey sauce evenly over the shrimp; then return to the oven and continue baking for 15 to 20 minutes, or until the shrimp are opaque and the sauce has formed a glaze. Serve hot.

SUBSTITUTION TIP: If you don't have shallots, you can use a small white or yellow onion instead.

PER SERVING: Total Calories: 184; Total Fat: 4g; Saturated Fat: 2g; Cholesterol: 221mg; Sodium: 399mg; Potassium: 24mg; Total Carbohydrate: 9g; Fiber: 0g; Sugars: 6g; Protein: 29g

SPICY PAN-FRIED RED SNAPPER

SERVES 4   **PREP TIME** 5 MINUTES   **COOK TIME** 12 MINUTES

Do you need a recipe for dinner in a flash without all the fuss? With just five ingredients, you can pull together a delicious, quick meal. Cajun seasoning—which combines paprika, garlic powder, onion powder, cayenne pepper, thyme, and oregano—adds a kick of flavor to this otherwise mild fish. Red snapper is a gout-friendly fish that goes well with baked potatoes, green beans, or roasted broccoli.

✓ **30-MINUTES**

✓ **DIABETIC FRIENDLY**

✓ **KIDNEY FRIENDLY**

✓ **ONE POT**

⅔ cup seasoned
  bread crumbs

1 teaspoon Cajun or
  seafood seasoning

1 pound red snapper fillets

1 tablespoon plus
  1 teaspoon olive or corn oil

1 lemon, cut into wedges

1. On a shallow plate, mix the bread crumbs and seasoning together. Dredge the snapper fillets in the seasoned bread crumbs to coat.

2. Heat the oil in a large skillet over medium heat.

3. Cook the coated snapper for 5 to 6 minutes per side, or until fish starts to flake. Serve with lemon wedges.

COOKING TIP: Red snapper can be broiled instead of fried. Place the broiler rack 5 inches from the cooking element. Place the coated fish on a broiler pan lined with parchment paper. Broil on high heat for 4 to 5 minutes per side.

PER SERVING: Total Calories: 173; Total Fat: 6g; Saturated Fat: 0g; Cholesterol: 0mg; Sodium: 193mg; Potassium: 0mg; Total Carbohydrate: 6g; Fiber: 0g; Sugars: 0g; Protein: 22g

PARCHMENT SALMON WITH LEMON

SERVES 4   **PREP TIME** 5 MINUTES   **COOK TIME** 15 MINUTES

If you've never used tarragon before, you're in for a treat. Tarragon has a licorice-like taste that goes well with fish and chicken dishes. This recipe is super simple for a weeknight meal but elegant enough for a fancy dinner. Salmon is known for its anti-inflammatory properties, making it a gout-friendly, heart-healthy food.

✓ **30-MINUTES**
✓ **DIABETIC FRIENDLY**
✓ **GLUTEN FREE**
✓ **KIDNEY FRIENDLY**
✓ **ONE POT**

Nonstick cooking spray

¼ cup olive oil

1 lemon, juiced
  (2 tablespoons)

2 teaspoons dried tarragon

½ teaspoon salt

4 (6-ounce) salmon
  fillets, skin on

1. Preheat the oven to 375°F. Line a 9-by-13-inch pan with parchment paper and spray it with nonstick spray.

2. In a medium bowl, whisk together the olive oil, lemon juice, tarragon, and salt. Add the salmon fillets, turning to coat them, and then place fillets in the lined baking pan.

3. Bake 10 to 15 minutes, or until the fish starts to flake.

4. Serve with buttered noodles, a baked potato, or roasted broccoli.

VARIATION TIP: Dried dill can be used in place of tarragon.

PER SERVING: Total Calories: 336; Total Fat: 23g; Saturated Fat: 3g; Cholesterol: 90mg; Sodium: 367mg; Potassium: 19mg; Total Carbohydrate: 0g; Fiber: 0g; Sugars: 0g; Protein: 33g

PARMESAN CRUSTED BROILED SCALLOPS

SERVES 4 **PREP TIME** 5 MINUTES **COOK TIME** 10 MINUTES

While scallops are slightly higher in purines than some other seafood, they can still be enjoyed in moderation (about three or four times a year). Scallops are a good source of protein and iodine—a nutrient that keeps your thyroid functioning normally. Grated Asiago cheese also works well in this recipe, if you don't have Parmesan.

✓ **30-MINUTES**
✓ **DIABETIC FRIENDLY**
✓ **KIDNEY FRIENDLY**
✓ **ONE POT**

⅓ cup Italian-seasoned bread crumbs

1 tablespoon grated Parmesan cheese

1 tablespoon fresh minced parsley

¼ teaspoon paprika

1½ pounds sea scallops

1 tablespoon butter, melted

1 lemon, cut into wedges

1. Line a broiler pan with foil or parchment paper and set it in the second rack position in the oven.

2. In a large resealable plastic bag, combine the bread crumbs, Parmesan cheese, parsley, and paprika. Brush the scallops with butter, and then add them to the bag. Seal and shake to coat.

3. Place the scallops on the broiler pan and broil 10 minutes, or until cooked through. Serve with lemon wedges.

TRIGGER TIP: Shrimp can be used in place of scallops if you'd like to enjoy this dish during a flare-up.

PER SERVING: Total Calories: 199; Total Fat: 5g; Saturated Fat: 2g;

Cholesterol: 65mg; Sodium: 390mg; Potassium: 567mg;

Total Carbohydrate: 7g; Fiber: 0g; Sugars: 0g; Protein: 30g

TUNA STEAKS WITH WASABI SAUCE

SERVES 6   **PREP TIME** 5 MINUTES   **COOK TIME** 35 MINUTES

Tuna can be eaten in moderation even if you have gout. Overall, tuna is lower in saturated fat and cholesterol than red meat, although it may be higher in purines. This recipe combines soy sauce, wasabi, and white wine to create a delicious dish that's a real crowd-pleaser.

✓ **30-MINUTES**
✓ **DIABETIC FRIENDLY**
✓ **GLUTEN-FREE**
✓ **KIDNEY FRIENDLY**
✓ **ONE POT**

10 ounces white wine or cooking sherry

2 tablespoons white wine vinegar

¼ cup minced onion

1 tablespoon wasabi paste

1 tablespoon low-sodium soy sauce

1 stick unsalted butter, cubed

½ cup olive oil plus 1 tablespoon, divided

1 cup cilantro leaves, chopped

6 (4 ounce) tuna steaks, 1-inch thick

½ teaspoon salt

½ teaspoon pepper

1. In a small saucepan over medium heat, combine the white wine, vinegar, and onion. Simmer until the liquid is reduced to about 2 tablespoons. Strain out the onions and discard, and then return the liquid to the pan.

2. Add the wasabi paste and soy sauce to the liquid. Slowly whisk in the butter and ½ cup of olive oil, making a smooth sauce. Add the cilantro; then remove from heat and set aside.

3. Brush tuna steaks with the remaining 1 tablespoon olive oil, and season with salt and pepper. In a large skillet, cook the tuna steaks over medium-high heat for 3 to 5 minutes on each side. The center of the tuna may still be a little pink. Serve tuna steaks with wasabi sauce.

TRIGGER TIP: If you prefer a fish lower in purines, you can use salmon in this dish instead of tuna.

SUBSTITUTION TIP: You can make this recipe alcohol-free by skipping the white wine and using low-sodium chicken broth instead.

PER SERVING: Total Calories: 303; Total Fat: 19g; Saturated Fat: 6g; Cholesterol: 63mg; Sodium: 434mg; Potassium: 76mg; Total Carbohydrate: 3g; Fiber: 0g; Sugars: 1g; Protein: 23g

FISH TACOS WITH PEACH SALSA

SERVES 4 **PREP TIME** 15 MINUTES, PLUS 15 MINUTES TO MARINATE **COOK TIME** 15 MINUTES

Tacos are not just made with beef! Fish tacos have become more popular on restaurant menus as consumers try to eat less red meat and add more seafood to their diets. Now you can make fish tacos yourself, paired with a delicious peach salsa.

✓ **30-MINUTES**
✓ **DIABETIC FRIENDLY**
✓ **GLUTEN-FREE**

3 tablespoons olive or corn oil

3 tablespoons lime juice

1 teaspoon ground cumin

1 garlic clove, minced

½ teaspoon salt

1 pound tilapia

2 peaches, chopped

¼ cup cilantro, chopped

¼ cup red onion, minced

½ jalapeño pepper, seeded and minced

½ teaspoon salt

8 corn tortillas

1. Whisk the olive oil, 2 tablespoons of the lime juice, cumin, garlic, and salt together in a large bowl. Add the tilapia and marinate for at least 15 minutes.

2. When ready to bake, preheat an oven to 400°F. Line a baking sheet with parchment paper or aluminum foil. Place the marinated fish on the baking pan and bake for 15 minutes.

3. Remove the fish from the oven and flake into small pieces.

4. While the fish is cooking, make the peach salsa. Combine the peaches, cilantro, red onion, jalapeño pepper, remaining lime juice, and salt.

5. Place a few tablespoons of flaked fish on each corn tortilla, and top with a tablespoon of peach salsa.

COOKING TIP: You can grill or blacken the fish in this recipe too. To grill, heat grill to medium-high heat and grill marinated fish for 10 to 15 minutes, or until done. For blackened fish, make a rub by combining 1 tablespoon of smoked paprika, ¾ teaspoon of onion powder, ½ teaspoon of salt, ¼ teaspoon pepper, ¼ teaspoon of dried thyme, ¼ teaspoon of dried oregano, and ⅛ teaspoon of cayenne pepper in a large bowl. Brush fish fillets with olive oil and then coat with blackened seasoning before baking.

PER SERVING: Total Calories: 330; Total Fat: 13g; Saturated Fat: 2g; Cholesterol: 55mg; Sodium: 645mg; Potassium: 282mg; Total Carbohydrate: 31g; Fiber: 5g; Sugars: 8g; Protein: 25g

SALMON WITH GINGER SOY MARINADE

SERVES 4   **PREP TIME** 15 MINUTES, PLUS 15 MINUTES TO MARINATE   **COOK TIME** 15 MINUTES

Did you know that salmon is not only good for your heart, it's also good for your waist? Salmon is one of the most filling varieties of fish, likely because of its healthy fat content. You'll love the simplicity and flavor of this recipe. Ginger paste is convenient to use and keeps in your fridge for months. Peanut oil also works well in place of sesame oil.

✓ **30-MINUTES**

✓ **DIABETIC FRIENDLY**

✓ **GLUTEN-FREE**

✓ **KIDNEY FRIENDLY**

✓ **ONE POT**

3 tablespoons canola oil

3 tablespoons rice wine vinegar or apple cider vinegar

2 tablespoons low-sodium soy sauce

1 tablespoon ginger paste

1 garlic clove, minced

1 teaspoon sesame oil

4 (4-ounce) salmon fillets

1 lemon cut into wedges (optional)

1. In a small bowl, whisk together the canola oil, vinegar, soy sauce, ginger paste, minced garlic, and sesame oil.

2. Place the salmon in a large resealable plastic bag and add the marinade. Massage the marinade into the fish. Refrigerate for a minimum of 15 minutes before grilling. The longer you marinate, the more intense the flavor.

3. Heat grill to medium-high heat when ready to cook the fish. Grill each piece for 5 to 7 minutes per side, or until the fish is cooked through. Serve with lemon wedges (if using).

COOKING TIP: Fish can be broiled instead of grilled. Place broiling rack 5 inches from heating element. Put the marinated salmon on a broiling pan lined with parchment paper and cook for 8 to 10 minutes, or until the fish is cooked through.

PER SERVING: Total Calories: 321; Total Fat: 24g; Saturated Fat: 4g; Cholesterol: 65mg; Sodium: 366mg; Potassium: 37mg; Total Carbohydrate: 2g; Fiber: 0g; Sugars: 0g; Protein: 23g

BROILED TILAPIA WITH HERBED MAYONNAISE

SERVES 4   **PREP TIME** 5 MINUTES   **COOK TIME** 10 MINUTES

It's important to get enough protein in your diet, and eating fish a few nights a week can help you achieve that goal. Tilapia is a versatile fish that's easy to cook and low in fat and sodium. Adding fresh and dried herbs, garlic, and lemon zest to mayonnaise gives it a deliciously different flavor without additional calories or fat.

✓ **30-MINUTE**

✓ **DIABETIC FRIENDLY**

✓ **GLUTEN-FREE**

1 small lemon

¼ cup olive oil mayonnaise or light mayonnaise

2 tablespoons fresh parsley

2 garlic cloves, minced

4 (4-ounce) tilapia fillets

½ teaspoon salt

½ teaspoon pepper

1. Preheat oven to broil and set the rack 5 inches below the broiling element. Line a baking sheet with aluminum foil or parchment paper and set aside.

2. Zest half the lemon for about 1 teaspoon of zest. Then cut the lemon into wedges for garnish.

3. In a small bowl, whisk together the mayonnaise, parsley, garlic, and lemon zest.

4. Pat the tilapia fillets dry with a paper towel and place them on the lined baking sheet. Season both sides of the tilapia with salt and pepper; then spread the mayonnaise mixture on the fillets.

5. Broil 6 to 8 minutes, or until the fish flakes easily with a fork and the top is golden brown. Garnish with lemon wedges.

SUBSTITUTION TIP: Dried parsley, tarragon, or dill can be substituted for fresh parsley if desired.

PER SERVING: Total Calories: 185; Total Fat: 7g; Saturated Fat: 2g; Cholesterol: 72mg; Sodium: 847mg; Potassium: 448mg; Total Carbohydrate: 2g; Fiber: 0g; Sugars: 0g; Protein: 30g

SIMPLE SHRIMP SCAMPI WITH ANGEL HAIR PASTA

SERVES 4   **PREP TIME** 10 MINUTES   **COOK TIME** 10 MINUTES

There's something irresistible about garlic, butter, and shrimp over pasta. It's no wonder it's often a featured favorite in Italian restaurants! This dish can be made for a weeknight meal or saved for a weekend to impress guests. If gluten is a concern, keep an eye out for gluten-free pasta.

✓ **30-MINUTE**
✓ **DIABETIC FRIENDLY**

1 pound angel hair pasta

2 tablespoons olive oil

1 pound baby shrimp, peeled and deveined

4 garlic cloves, minced

½ teaspoon red pepper flakes

½ cup dry white wine

1 lemon, juiced

4 tablespoons butter

1 teaspoon lemon zest

¼ cup fresh parsley leaves, chopped

1. Bring a large pot of water to a boil, add the pasta, and cook for 8 minutes, or until al dente. Drain and set aside.

2. While the pasta is cooking, heat a large skillet over medium heat and add the olive oil. Once the skillet is hot, add the shrimp and cook for 2 to 3 minutes. Remove from the pan and set aside.

3. Combine the garlic and red pepper flakes to the skillet and sauté for 1 minute. Add the white wine and lemon juice. Increase the heat and let the liquid reduce slightly. Whisk in the butter and add the shrimp back in. Cook for 2 to 3 minutes, or until heated through.

4. Add the cooked shrimp, lemon zest, and parsley to the cooked pasta and serve.

VARIATION: To add color, texture, and nutrition, sauté 4 cups of baby spinach leaves along with the garlic and add it to the pasta. This adds beta-carotene, vitamin C, and potassium to the dish.

PER SERVING: Total Calories: 725; Total Fat: 22g; Saturated Fat: 9g; Cholesterol: 252mg; Sodium: 347mg; Potassium: 525mg; Total Carbohydrate: 87g; Fiber: 4g; Sugars: 3g; Protein: 39g

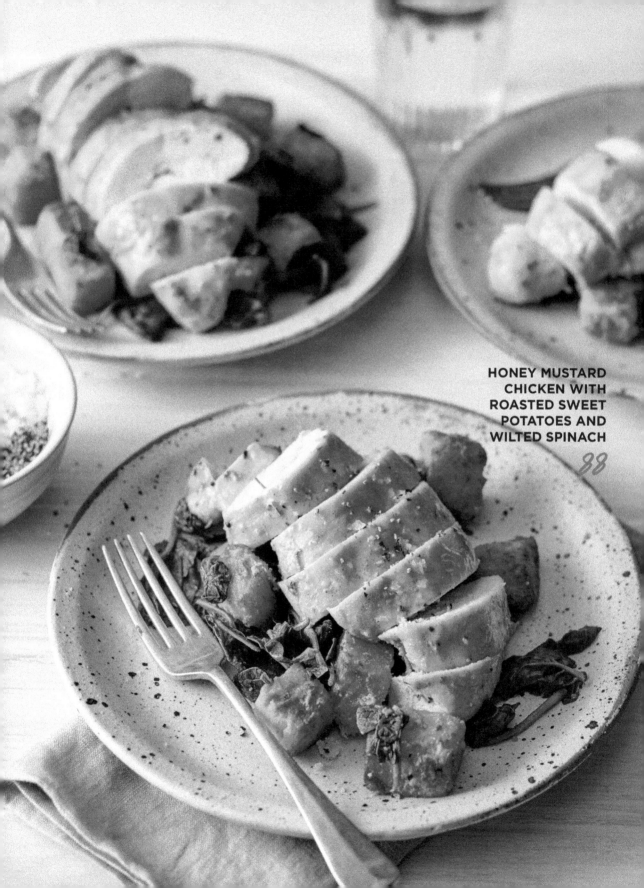

**HONEY MUSTARD
CHICKEN WITH
ROASTED SWEET
POTATOES AND
WILTED SPINACH**

88

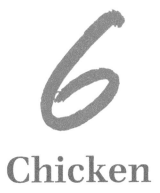

Chicken

Chicken is one of the most versatile sources of protein but is often thought of as boring or something you prepare when you can't think of anything else. This chapter will change that! I've collected recipes that are easy to prepare and have flavors that are fun to experiment with. You'll find delicious, complete meals such as Dijon Chicken with Green Beans and Farro (page 80), Pasta Primavera with Blackened Chicken (page 81), and Pesto Chicken with Broccoli (page 85).

DIJON CHICKEN WITH GREEN BEANS AND FARRO

SERVES 4 **PREP TIME** 5 MINUTES **COOK TIME** 20 MINUTES

Skinless chicken breast is a safe and healthy choice when it comes to managing gout. It's low in purines as well as saturated fat and cholesterol. Green beans are a source of vitamin C, an antioxidant that's important for a strong immune system. Farro— a high-fiber, high-protein ancient grain that's related to modern-day wheat—has a nutty flavor and pairs well with the tangy taste of Dijon mustard.

✓ **30-MINUTE**

✓ **DIABETIC FRIENDLY**

3 cups water plus
  2 tablespoons, divided

1 cup farro

3 tablespoons extra-virgin
  olive oil, divided

1 lb. boneless, skinless
  chicken breast

1 teaspoon salt, divided

2 cups frozen green beans

3 green onions, thinly sliced
  (white and green parts)

2 tablespoons white
  wine vinegar

1 tablespoon dried oregano

1 teaspoon Dijon mustard

2 tablespoons minced onion

1. In a medium pot, bring 3 cups of water to a boil. Add farro and cook for 5 minutes; then reduce the heat and cook about 20 minutes, or until farro is tender. Drain and set aside to cool.

2. While the farro is cooking, heat 1 tablespoon of olive oil in a skillet. Sprinkle the chicken with ½ teaspoon of salt and cook for 8 minutes on each side. Let cool, and then cut into ½-inch cubes.

3. Place the green beans and the remaining 2 tablespoons of water in a microwave-safe bowl. Microwave for 3 minutes, and then set aside.

4. Mix the farro, chicken, and green beans in a large bowl. Add the green onions.

5. In a small bowl, whisk together the remaining 2 tablespoons of olive oil, vinegar, oregano, mustard, and remaining ½ teaspoon of salt. Add the minced onion.

6. Pour the dressing over the chicken and vegetables and toss to coat. This dish can be served warm, or chilled for 1 hour and served cold.

SUBSTITUTION TIP: Use quinoa or brown rice if you'd like to make the recipe gluten-free.

PER SERVING: Total Calories: 378; Total Fat: 15g; Saturated Fat: 2g; Cholesterol: 73mg; Sodium: 659mg; Potassium: 599mg; Total Carbohydrate: 30g; Fiber: 7g; Sugars: 1g; Protein: 30g

PASTA PRIMAVERA WITH BLACKENED CHICKEN

SERVES 4   **PREP TIME** 15 MINUTES   **COOK TIME** 15 MINUTES

Primavera means "spring" in Italian, but you can make this dish any time of year. A variety of vegetables provide antioxidants, vitamin C, beta-carotene, and fiber—plus color and flavor. Using whole-wheat noodles adds more fiber without compromising flavor.

✓ **30-MINUTE**

✓ **DIABETIC FRIENDLY**

8 ounces whole-wheat penne or rotini

2 chicken breasts (about 1 pound), cut into ½-inch pieces

2 teaspoons Cajun seasoning

1 tablespoon olive oil

1 tablespoon butter

3 garlic cloves, minced

½ red bell pepper, chopped

½ yellow bell pepper, chopped

½ red onion, diced

10 asparagus stalks, woody ends trimmed, cut into 1-inch pieces

½ cup frozen peas

½ cup half-and-half

Shredded Parmesan cheese, for serving

Salt, for serving

Freshly ground pepper, for serving

1. Bring a large pot of water to a boil. Add the pasta and cook 8 to 9 minutes, or until al dente. Drain and set aside in a large bowl.

2. While the pasta is cooking, place the chicken in a small bowl with the Cajun seasoning and toss to coat.

3. Heat the olive oil in a large skillet over medium heat. Add the seasoned chicken and cook for 4 to 5 minutes per side, or until cooked through. Remove from skillet and set aside.

4. In the same skillet, add the butter, garlic, bell pepper, onion, asparagus, and peas and sauté for 2 minutes. The vegetables should still be still bright in color, soft but not soggy.

5. Add the half-and-half and reserved chicken, and cook for 2 to 4 minutes, or until sauce has thickened slightly.

6. Add the vegetable mixture to the cooked pasta and toss to coat. Serve with the shredded Parmesan cheese, salt, and freshly ground pepper.

TRIGGER TIP: Saturated fat can be reduced further by using all olive oil instead of butter, and whole milk instead of half-and-half. You can also omit the Parmesan cheese.

PER SERVING: Total Calories: 425; Total Fat: 12g; Saturated Fat: 5g; Cholesterol: 59mg; Sodium: 122mg; Potassium: 355mg; Total Carbohydrate: 52g; Fiber: 5g; Sugars: 5g; Protein: 27g

SPICY CHICKEN WITH CHICKPEAS

SERVES 6 **PREP TIME** 15 MINUTES, PLUS 60 MINUTES TO MARINATE **COOK TIME** 30 MINUTES

This recipe couldn't be simpler or more packed with flavor. Chicken thighs and chickpeas are nicely spiced with paprika, garlic, and cumin and then roasted all together in one pan for easy cleanup. This is a high-protein, high-fiber dish that can be paired with whole-grain couscous or a big green salad if you're trying to limit carbohydrates.

✓ DIABETIC FRIENDLY

✓ GLUTEN-FREE

✓ ONE POT

⅓ cup olive oil

4 garlic cloves, chopped

½ cup chopped cilantro, plus more for garnish

2 teaspoons smoked paprika

1½ teaspoons ground cumin

½ teaspoon crushed red pepper flakes

2 teaspoons sea salt

1 teaspoon freshly ground black pepper

4 chicken thighs, fat trimmed

2 (15-ounce) cans chickpeas, drained and rinsed

2 pints cherry tomatoes

1. In a large bowl, combine the olive oil, garlic, cilantro, paprika, cumin, red pepper flakes, salt, and black pepper. Add the chicken, chickpeas, and tomatoes, and toss to coat. Cover the bowl and marinate for at least 1 hour but no more than 24 hours.

2. When ready to cook, preheat the oven to 450°F. Line a large baking pan with parchment paper and spread out the marinated chicken mixture evenly on the pan.

3. Roast for 30 to 35 minutes, or until the chicken is browned and cooked through. Garnish with additional cilantro and serve with rice, couscous, or salad.

VARIATION TIP: To change up the flavor of this dish, try using fresh parsley instead of cilantro.

PER SERVING: Total Calories: 421; Total Fat: 25g; Saturated Fat: 5g; Cholesterol: 63mg; Sodium: 595mg; Potassium: 561mg; Total Carbohydrate: 29g; Fiber: 8g; Sugars: 7g; Protein: 22g

CHICKEN FAJITAS

SERVES 6   **PREP TIME** 10 MINUTES, PLUS 30 MINUTES TO MARINATE   **COOK TIME** 20 MINUTES

The term *fajita* originally referred to skirt steak, but this Tex-Mex favorite has branched out to include chicken, shrimp, and even tofu. Peppers and onions are traditionally combined with your choice of protein, but I've found that using zucchini, eggplant, or other vegetables can be equally tasty. Using whole-wheat or corn tortillas boosts the fiber of this antioxidant-rich dish too.

✓ **30-MINUTE**
✓ **DIABETIC FRIENDLY**
✓ **KIDNEY FRIENDLY**

½ cup plus 1 tablespoon
  corn or vegetable
  oil, divided

3 limes, juiced (¼ cup)

2 garlic cloves, minced

2 teaspoons ground cumin

½ teaspoon crushed red
  pepper flakes

½ teaspoon salt

1 teaspoon freshly ground
  black pepper

3 chicken breasts

1 red or yellow bell pepper,
  cut into strips

1 green bell pepper, cut
  into strips

1 large red onion, sliced

6 large whole-wheat tortillas
  or 12 small corn tortillas

1. In a large bowl, whisk together ½ cup of corn oil, lime juice, garlic, cumin, crushed red pepper flakes, salt, and pepper. Add the chicken and toss to coat. Marinate the chicken for at least 30 minutes, and up to 2 hours.

2. Heat the remaining 1 tablespoon of oil in a large skillet when ready to cook the chicken. Cook the chicken for 8 to 10 minutes per side, or until done. Set the chicken aside to rest for about 10 minutes, and then slice it into strips.

3. Add bell peppers and onions to the same skillet, and cook for 5 minutes, or until soft. Add the cooked chicken strips back to the skillet and cook to heat through, about 3 minutes. Serve with the tortillas.

SUBSTITUTION TIP: Lemon juice may be used if you don't have limes.

PER SERVING: Total Calories: 243; Total Fat: 8g; Saturated Fat: 1g; Cholesterol: 43mg; Sodium: 439mg; Potassium: 196mg; Total Carbohydrate: 22g; Fiber: 2g; Sugars: 3g; Protein: 21g

PEANUT NOODLES WITH CHICKEN

SERVES 6   **PREP TIME** 10 MINUTES   **COOK TIME** 15 MINUTES

Tired of the same old chicken? Try something nutty! This recipe, inspired by traditional pad Thai, can be whipped up in a flash and uses peanut butter as an easy, low-purine boost of flavor. To make the meal more kid-friendly, skip the red pepper flakes, cilantro, and green onions.

✓ **30-MINUTE**

✓ **DIABETIC FRIENDLY**

1 pound
 whole-wheat spaghetti

1 tablespoon canola oil

1 medium red or yellow bell
 pepper, cut into strips

¾ cup water

½ cup peanut butter
 (smooth or crunchy)

3 tablespoons low-sodium
 soy sauce

1½ teaspoon ginger paste

1 garlic clove, minced

1 to 2 teaspoons crushed
 red pepper flakes

2 cups cooked chicken
 (can use rotisserie chicken
 or canned chicken)

3 green onions,
 sliced diagonally

½ cup chopped cilantro

1. Bring a large pot of water to a boil. Add the pasta and cook for 8 to 9 minutes, or until al dente. Drain and set aside in a large bowl.

2. While the pasta is cooking, heat canola oil in a skillet. Add the peppers and sauté for 5 minutes, or until softened; then add to pasta.

3. In a medium saucepan, whisk together the water, peanut butter, soy sauce, ginger paste, garlic, and red pepper flakes. Simmer over medium-low heat for 5 minutes, or until the sauce is creamy. More water can be added to thin the sauce if needed.

4. Add the chicken to the pasta and peppers. Pour peanut sauce over the pasta and toss to coat. Sprinkle the green onions and chopped cilantro on top and serve hot.

VARIATION TIP: This dish can be made gluten-free by using rice noodles and omitting the soy sauce. You can also use liquid aminos in place of soy sauce.

PER SERVING: Total Calories: 497; Total Fat: 16g; Saturated Fat: 3g; Cholesterol: 36mg; Sodium: 437mg; Potassium: 484mg; Total Carbohydrate: 64g; Fiber: 2g; Sugars: 3g; Protein: 31g

PESTO CHICKEN WITH BROCCOLI

SERVES 6 **PREP TIME** 5 MINUTES **COOK TIME** 25 MINUTES

This recipe can be made using any leftover chicken and pasta or started from scratch. All you'll need is olive oil, pesto, garlic, and broccoli. Broccoli is a great addition to any meal because it adds anti-inflammatory phytochemicals, fiber, and a burst of color. Use whole-grain pasta to increase the fiber content and enhance the texture.

✓ **30-MINUTE**

✓ **DIABETIC FRIENDLY**

16 ounces whole-wheat penne or shell noodles

2 large chicken breasts

½ teaspoon salt

½ teaspoon pepper

4 tablespoons olive oil, divided

2 garlic cloves, minced

1 broccoli head cut into 2-inch florets

2 tablespoons jarred pesto

¼ cup Parmesan cheese (optional)

1. Bring a large pot of water to a boil and add the pasta. Cook for 8 to 10 minutes, or until al dente. Drain and set aside in a large bowl.

2. While the pasta is cooking, season the chicken with salt and pepper, and then cut it into 1-inch pieces.

3. Heat 2 tablespoons of olive oil in a large skillet and add the chicken pieces. Cook for 10 to 12 minutes, stirring, or until cooked through. Add the garlic and cook for 1 more minute.

4. While the chicken is cooking, place the broccoli in a microwave-safe bowl. Cover and microwave for 4 minutes. Once the broccoli is done, add the broccoli and chicken to the pasta.

5. In a small bowl, whisk together the remaining 2 tablespoons of olive oil and the pesto. Add to the pasta and chicken and toss to coat. Serve with shredded Parmesan cheese (if using).

VARIATION TIP: Sundried tomato pesto can be used in place of traditional pesto for a change in flavor.

PER SERVING: Total Calories: 433; Total Fat: 11g; Saturated Fat: 1g; Cholesterol: 34mg; Sodium: 322mg; Potassium: 246mg; Total Carbohydrate: 57g; Fiber: 8g; Sugars: 4g; Protein: 29g

COCONUT SPICE CHICKEN IN PITA

SERVES 4 **PREP TIME** 5 MINUTES **COOK TIME** 20 MINUTES

This gout-friendly, low-fat recipe combines plain yogurt, ginger, garlic, and a few aromatic spices to create a dish you'll want to make over and over again. I usually use this chicken in a pita sandwich with fresh spinach, cucumbers, and tomatoes to boost the antioxidant content. It can also be served over rice or a big green salad.

✓ **30-MINUTE**
✓ **DIABETIC FRIENDLY**
✓ **ONE POT**

¾ cup plain, low-fat yogurt

½ cup shredded coconut

1 tablespoon ginger paste

2 garlic cloves, minced

¾ teaspoon salt

½ teaspoon ground cumin

½ teaspoon
  ground coriander

¼ teaspoon cayenne pepper

1 pound chicken tenderloins

2 whole-wheat pitas,
  cut in half

2 cups fresh baby
  spinach leaves

½ cucumber, chopped

12 cherry tomatoes, halved

1 tablespoon olive oil

1. Turn the oven to broil and place the oven rack 6 inches away from the broiler element. Line a broiling pan with parchment paper.

2. In a medium mixing bowl, mix the yogurt, coconut, ginger paste, garlic, salt, cumin, coriander, and cayenne pepper. Dredge each piece of chicken in the yogurt mixture until fully coated.

3. Place the chicken on the broiling pan and broil for 10 minutes. Once it has started to brown, flip the chicken over and broil for another 10 minutes, or until cooked through.

4. Place 2 chicken tenderloins in a pita pocket with ½ cup of spinach leaves, 2 tablespoons of chopped cucumbers, and 6 tomato halves. Repeat to make 3 more pitas. Drizzle with olive oil and serve.

COOKING TIP: Chicken may also be grilled. Cover the grill grate with aluminum foil and grill chicken for 20 minutes, flipping chicken tenders every 5 minutes. Double or even triple the recipe to feed a larger crowd.

PER SERVING: Total Calories: 301; Total Fat: 8g; Saturated Fat: 3g; Cholesterol: 67mg; Sodium: 722mg; Potassium: 435mg; Total Carbohydrate: 26g; Fiber: 4g; Sugars: 5g; Protein: 33g

CHICKEN WITH FRESH FENNEL AND LEMON ORZO

SERVES 4   **PREP TIME** 5 MINUTES   **COOK TIME** 25 MINUTES

The flavors in this dish may sound somewhat unconventional at first, but everyone who tries it loves how they taste together. I use garlic, fennel, and leeks, all of which have anti-inflammatory properties. Grated lemon zest gives the orzo a refreshing twist in addition to providing antioxidants.

✓ **30-MINUTE**

✓ **DIABETIC FRIENDLY**

✓ **ONE POT**

6 boneless skinless chicken breasts

½ teaspoon sea salt

½ teaspoon freshly ground black pepper

2 tablespoons olive oil

1 tablespoon butter

1 fennel bulb, chopped

1 leek, chopped (white and green parts)

8 ounces orzo

2½ cups low-sodium chicken broth

⅓ cup white wine

1 tablespoon fresh lemon juice

1 teaspoon grated lemon zest

¼ cup fresh parsley, chopped

1. Season the chicken with salt and pepper.

2. Heat the olive oil in a Dutch oven or large pot over medium heat. Add the chicken breasts and cook for 6 to 8 minutes, or until browned on both sides. Add the butter, fennel, and leek to the skillet and cook for 5 minutes. Add the orzo and cook for 3 minutes.

3. Pour in chicken broth, white wine, and lemon juice, and simmer on medium heat for 20 to 25 minutes, or until the orzo and chicken are fully cooked. Top with the lemon zest and chopped parsley prior to serving.

VARIATION TIP: Chopped rosemary can replace the parsley to give the dish a different flavor.

SUBSTITUTION TIP: To make this recipe alcohol-free, you can replace the white wine with ⅓ cup of white grape juice and ½ teaspoon of lemon juice.

PER SERVING: Total Calories: 566; Total Fat: 14g; Saturated Fat: 3g; Cholesterol: 121mg; Sodium: 468mg; Potassium: 333mg; Total Carbohydrate: 51g; Fiber: 4g; Sugars: 4g; Protein: 55g

HONEY MUSTARD CHICKEN WITH ROASTED SWEET POTATOES AND WILTED SPINACH

SERVES 4   **PREP TIME** 15 MINUTES   **COOK TIME** 45 MINUTES

Looking for a one-dish meal that tastes great, one everyone will enjoy that has something a little different for your palate? I've got you covered! Cinnamon is loaded with antioxidants, has anti-inflammatory properties, and adds a touch of spice to sweet potatoes. Spinach provides a dose of potassium and iron and is also a great source of beta-carotene and vitamins A, C, and K.

✓ **DIABETIC FRIENDLY**

✓ **GLUTEN-FREE**

✓ **ONE POT**

4 boneless skinless chicken breasts

½ teaspoon salt

½ teaspoon pepper

½ cup honey

½ cup Dijon mustard

1 teaspoon dried rosemary

½ teaspoon paprika

2 large sweet potatoes, peeled and cubed

½ teaspoon ground cinnamon

1 (10-ounce) bag fresh spinach

1. Preheat the oven to 350°F. Line a 9-by-13-inch baking dish with parchment paper.

2. Season the chicken with salt and pepper, and then place on one side of the baking dish.

3. In a small bowl, whisk together the honey, mustard, rosemary, and paprika. Pour the mustard sauce over the chicken.

4. Dust the sweet potatoes with cinnamon and place them on the other side of the baking dish.

5. Spread the spinach evenly over the chicken and sweet potatoes. Bake for 30 minutes, or until chicken and potatoes are fully cooked.

SUBSTITUTION TIP: Stone-ground mustard can be used in place of Dijon mustard for a slightly different flavor.

PER SERVING: Total Calories: 345; Total Fat: 3g; Saturated Fat: 0g; Cholesterol: 65mg; Sodium: 814mg; Potassium: 683mg; Total Carbohydrate: 53g; Fiber: 5g; Sugars: 38g; Protein: 31g

CHICKEN TIKKA MASALA

SERVES 4   **PREP TIME** 15 MINUTES   **COOK TIME** 45 MINUTES

While this recipe may look intimidating at first glance, don't let it scare you. You likely already have some of these ingredients on hand. In addition to being a tasty, restaurant-quality dinner, this recipe provides a bit of calcium and protein from the yogurt, which is beneficial to those dealing with gout. Cayenne pepper provides a little kick to the dish but can be left out to turn down the spice level.

✓ **DIABETIC FRIENDLY**

✓ **GLUTEN-FREE**

✓ **ONE POT**

1 cup plain low-fat or fat-free yogurt

1 tablespoon lemon juice

1 tablespoon ginger paste

4 teaspoons ground cumin, divided

2 teaspoons cayenne pepper

2 teaspoons freshly ground black pepper

1 teaspoon ground cinnamon

2 teaspoons salt, divided

3 boneless chicken breasts, cut into ½-inch chunks

1 tablespoon butter

1 garlic clove, minced

2 teaspoons paprika

1 cup half-and-half

1 (8-ounce) can tomato sauce

½ cup fresh cilantro, chopped

1. Preheat the oven to 400°F. Line a 9-by-13-inch baking pan with aluminum foil.

2. In a medium bowl, stir together the yogurt, lemon juice, ginger paste, 2 teaspoons of cumin, cayenne pepper, black pepper, cinnamon, and 1 teaspoon of salt. Add the chicken and toss to coat.

3. Place the chicken on the baking pan and cook 30 minutes, or until done. Remove from oven and set aside.

4. While the chicken is cooking, melt the butter in a Dutch oven or large skillet. Add the remaining 2 teaspoons of cumin, remaining 1 teaspoon of salt, garlic, and paprika, and sauté for 3 minutes.

5. Add the half-and-half and tomato sauce to the skillet and simmer for 3 to 5 minutes, or until sauce thickens slightly. Add the cooked chicken and simmer on low heat for 10 minutes. Garnish with fresh cilantro and serve over rice or with naan.

TRIGGER TIP: Add 2 teaspoons of curry powder in place of cayenne pepper to provide more anti-inflammatory spice to the dish.

PER SERVING: Total Calories: 297; Total Fat: 13g; Saturated Fat: 6g; Cholesterol: 96mg; Sodium: 1634mg; Potassium: 556mg; Total Carbohydrate: 15g; Fiber: 3g; Sugars: 8g; Protein: 33g

BALSAMIC MARINATED CHICKEN

SERVES 4   **PREP TIME** 10 MINUTES, PLUS 30 MINUTES TO MARINATE   **COOK TIME** 10 MINUTES

I guarantee that this balsamic mixture will become your go-to chicken marinade. It's ready in a flash, tastes amazing, and uses simple spices like oregano, salt, and pepper. Anti-inflammatory garlic, rosemary, and olive oil also give this savory chicken great flavor. It can be grilled outside during warm months and broiled when it's cooler outside.

✓ **30-MINUTE**
✓ **DIABETIC FRIENDLY**
✓ **GLUTEN-FREE**
✓ **KIDNEY FRIENDLY**
✓ **ONE POT**

½ cup olive oil

¼ cup balsamic vinegar

2 lemons, juiced (¼ cup)

4 garlic cloves, minced

1 tablespoon dried rosemary

1 tablespoon dried oregano

2 teaspoons kosher or
  sea salt

1 teaspoon freshly ground
  black pepper

4 boneless chicken
  breasts, butterflied (slice
  horizontally to cut in half)

Nonstick cooking spray

1. In a large bowl or large resealable plastic bag, combine the olive oil, vinegar, lemon juice, garlic, rosemary, oregano, salt, and pepper. Add the chicken breasts and toss to coat. Marinate the chicken for at least 20 minutes and up to 6 hours.

2. Spray your grill with nonstick cooking spray and then preheat to 375°F.

3. Place the marinated chicken on the grill and grill for 4 to 5 minutes per side, or until the chicken is fully cooked. Remove the chicken from the grill and allow it to rest for 5 minutes before serving.

COOKING TIP: Chicken can be cooked on the stovetop using a grill pan. Spray a grill pan with nonstick cooking spray, add the chicken, and cook 4 to 5 minutes per side, or until fully cooked.

PER SERVING: Total Calories: 366; Total Fat: 27g; Saturated Fat: 4g; Cholesterol: 65mg; Sodium: 1019mg; Potassium: 82mg; Total Carbohydrate: 6g; Fiber: 1g; Sugars: 3g; Protein: 27g

GARLIC PARMESAN CHICKEN WITH FRESH PARSLEY

SERVES 6   **PREP TIME** 10 MINUTES   **COOK TIME** 15 MINUTES

Is there any better combination than garlic and Parmesan cheese? Actually, yes! Adding fresh parsley brings flavor, color, and antioxidants to this delightful chicken recipe. This dish is also loaded with mushrooms and tomatoes, which add texture, color, and additional nutritional benefits, including vitamin C and fiber.

✓ **30-MINUTE**
✓ **DIABETIC FRIENDLY**
✓ **KIDNEY FRIENDLY**
✓ **ONE POT**

½ cup all-purpose flour

½ teaspoon salt

½ teaspoon pepper

3 boneless chicken breasts, sliced in half lengthwise

3 tablespoons olive oil, divided

2 cups button mushrooms, chopped

½ cup low-sodium chicken broth

1 large tomato, seeded and chopped

6 garlic cloves, minced

¼ cup fresh parsley, chopped

2 tablespoons butter

¼ cup grated Parmesan cheese

1. Place the flour, salt, and pepper in a large bowl or large resealable plastic bag. Add the chicken and toss to coat.

2. In a large skillet, heat 2 tablespoons of olive oil over medium heat. Add the chicken and cook 5 minutes per side, or until cooked through. Remove the chicken from the pan and set aside.

3. Heat the remaining 1 tablespoon of olive oil in the skillet. Add the mushrooms and cook for 3 to 4 minutes, until they have released their liquid.

4. Add the chicken broth, tomato, garlic, parsley, and butter. Stir until the butter is melted. Add the chicken back to the pan and cook for 3 to 5 minutes, until heated through. Sprinkle the chicken with the Parmesan cheese and serve.

VARIATION TIP: If you're not a mushroom fan, try asparagus or bell peppers instead.

PER SERVING: Total Calories: 244; Total Fat: 13g; Saturated Fat: 4g; Cholesterol: 57mg; Sodium: 325mg; Potassium: 187mg; Total Carbohydrate: 11g; Fiber: 1g; Sugars: 1g; Protein: 21g

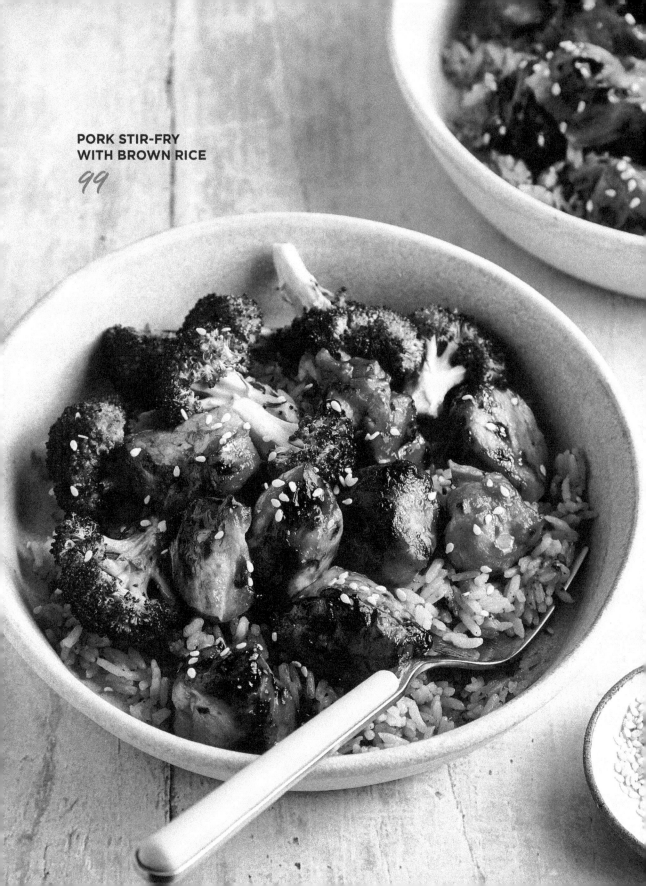

**PORK STIR-FRY
WITH BROWN RICE**
99

7

Beef and Pork

Red meat may be higher in purines, but that doesn't mean you can never eat it. In this chapter, you'll pick up tips about which cuts of beef and pork are best for preventing gout flare-ups as well as various ways to prepare them to reduce inflammation. Enjoy recipes like Pork Carnitas (page 102), Beef Tenderloin in Coffee Marinade (page 100), and Garlic Rosemary Roasted Pork Tenderloin (page 103).

SAVORY ROSEMARY MARINATED FLANK STEAK

SERVES 6 **PREP TIME** 45 MINUTES, 20 TO 30 MINUTES MARINADE TIME
COOK TIME 15 MINUTES

This is sure to be your new go-to steak recipe! While fattier cuts of red meat should be limited during a gout flare-up, using a lean cut such as flank steak will keep the saturated fat content lower. Because this recipe uses red meat, I consciously worked to keep the fat content low and used corn oil, a heart-healthy fat that lowers your LDL ("bad") cholesterol.

✓ **DIABETIC FRIENDLY**
✓ **ONE POT**

¼ cup corn oil

¼ cup apple cider vinegar

¼ cup low-sodium soy sauce

1 tablespoon yellow mustard

1 tablespoon dried rosemary

1 teaspoon salt

½ teaspoon freshly ground
  black pepper

½ yellow onion, chopped

3 garlic cloves, minced

1½ pounds flank steak

1. In a small bowl, whisk together the oil, vinegar, soy sauce, mustard, rosemary, salt, and pepper. Stir in the onions and garlic.

2. Place the steak in a large resealable plastic bag. Pour marinade into the bag and place in the refrigerator. Marinate for at least 30 minutes and no more than 2 days.

3. Preheat the grill to medium-high heat. Remove the flank steak from the marinade, reserving a few tablespoons of marinade to baste the steak later.

4. Cook the steak for 6 to 8 minutes, or until firm and hot in the center, brushing the steak occasionally with extra marinade. Once the steak has cooked through (its internal temperature should read 150°F), remove it from the grill and place on a cutting board. Allow the steak to rest for 5 minutes; then slice on the grain and serve.

VARIATION TIP: Substitute balsamic vinegar for the apple cider vinegar for a stronger flavor.

COOKING TIP: Steak may also be cooked on the stovetop using a large skillet. Coat a skillet with nonstick spray and cook the steak for 5 to 7 minutes per side, or until cooked through.

PER SERVING: Total Calories: 199; Total Fat: 9g; Saturated Fat: 3g; Cholesterol: 50mg; Sodium: 553mg; Potassium: 29mg; Total Carbohydrate: 2g; Fiber: 0g; Sugars: 1g; Protein: 25g

ROPA VIEJA (Flank Steak Simmered with Tomatoes and Peppers)

SERVES 6   **PREP TIME** 10 MINUTES   **COOK TIME** 25 MINUTES

You'll love this delicious Cuban dish! It's quick to prepare and has a whole lot of nutritional value. Chock-full of vitamin C from the stewed tomatoes and bell peppers, this meal has a real flavorful punch. Cumin, onions, and garlic provide flavor and anti-inflammatory properties. It can be made in a slow cooker while you're out or prepared on the stovetop in a large stockpot.

✓ **DIABETIC FRIENDLY**

✓ **GLUTEN-FREE**

✓ **ONE POT**

1 tablespoon corn oil

2 pounds flank or skirt steak

1 cup low-sodium
  beef broth

1 (8-ounce) can
  tomato sauce

1 (6-ounce) can
  tomato paste

1 small white or yellow
  onion, sliced

1 green or yellow bell
  pepper, cut into strips

2 garlic cloves, minced

1 tablespoon white vinegar

1 teaspoon ground cumin

12 mini corn or flour tortillas

2 teaspoons fresh
  cilantro, chopped

1. Heat the oil in a medium skillet. Add the steak and cook 3 minutes per side, or until browned; then set aside.

2. In a slow cooker, combine the beef broth, tomato sauce, tomato paste, onion, bell pepper, garlic, vinegar, and cumin. Add the steak and cook on low heat for 6 to 8 hours, or until the steak shreds easily with a fork.

3. Shred the steak with two forks. Place a few tablespoons of steak into a tortilla with a pinch of chopped cilantro. Fold over and enjoy!

COOKING TIP: To cook on the stove, add all the sauce ingredients to a large pot. Add the browned steak and simmer over low heat for 30 to 40 minutes. Shred the steak and use in tacos or over rice.

PER SERVING: Total Calories: 396; Total Fat: 13g; Saturated Fat: 5g; Cholesterol: 67mg; Sodium: 336mg; Potassium: 566mg; Total Carbohydrate: 31g; Fiber: 5g; Sugars: 7g; Protein: 38g

BLACK PEPPERCORN PORK

SERVES 6   **PREP TIME** 60 MINUTES, 20 TO 30 MINUTES MARINADE TIME
COOK TIME 25 MINUTES

This pork recipe may be simple to prepare, but the flavor really pops. Fresh black peppercorn, garlic, and rosemary complement one another perfectly. Use a lean cut of pork, such as tenderloin, to keep the purine content, saturated fat, and cholesterol count lower in your meal. This marinade would also go well with your favorite cut of lean beef. Serve with a big leafy green salad and a whole grain like quinoa or brown rice.

✓ **DIABETIC FRIENDLY**
✓ **GLUTEN-FREE**
✓ **KIDNEY FRIENDLY**
✓ **ONE POT**

½ cup fresh lemon juice

½ cup extra-virgin olive oil

4 garlic cloves, minced

2 tablespoons
 dried rosemary

2 tablespoons cracked
 black peppercorns

1 tablespoon kosher salt

1 pound pork tenderloin,
 visible fat trimmed

1. Preheat the grill to 450°F.

2. In a large resealable plastic bag, combine the lemon juice, oil, garlic, rosemary, peppercorns, and salt. Add the pork and marinate for at least 1 hour.

3. Place the pork on the grill and close the lid. Grill the pork for 5 minutes; then rotate meat every 5 minutes, or until pork is no longer pink or an internal temperature of 145°F is reached.

4. To broil the pork instead, preheat the broiler and set the oven rack 5 inches below the broiler element. Place the pork tenderloin on a broiling pan and broil for 5 minutes; then turn and continue to broil for 5 minutes per side, or until cooked through.

5. Slice pork into 1-inch medallions and serve hot.

TRIGGER TIP: This marinade is also great with chicken or salmon.

PER SERVING: Total Calories: 123; Total Fat: 7g; Saturated Fat: 2g; Cholesterol: 43mg; Sodium: 432mg; Potassium: 10mg; Total Carbohydrate: 0g; Fiber: 0g; Sugars: 0g; Protein: 13g

CHILI LIME STEAK

SERVES 4 **PREP TIME** 20 MINUTES, 20 TO 30 MINUTES MARINADE TIME
COOK TIME 15 MINUTES

Lean red meat can be enjoyed in moderation for most people who are prone to gout. Marinating steak in an acidic medium (such as vinegar or citrus juice) helps tenderize the steak and gives it a tangy flavor. It also helps reduce the cancer-causing compounds that are produced when meat is grilled or broiled. Flank steak can be grilled, broiled, or cooked on the stove. This lean steak can be served over a big leafy salad or accompanied by mashed sweet potatoes.

✓ **DIABETIC FRIENDLY**
✓ **GLUTEN-FREE**
✓ **KIDNEY FRIENDLY**

2 tablespoons lime juice

1 tablespoon apple cider vinegar

1 teaspoon ground cumin

1 teaspoon chili powder

1 teaspoon onion powder

1 teaspoon salt

¼ teaspoon freshly ground black pepper

1 pound flank steak

Nonstick cooking spray

1. In a large bowl, whisk together the lime juice, vinegar, cumin, chili powder, onion powder, salt, and black pepper.

2. Trim visible fat from the flank steak and score with a fork along the natural grooves in the steak.

3. Add the flank steak to the bowl and refrigerate. Marinate for a minimum of 20 to 30 minutes but not longer than 24 hours.

4. When ready to broil the steak, preheat the broiler. Place the oven rack a few inches below the broiler element. Line a broiler pan with aluminum foil, and then spray the foil with nonstick cooking spray. Place the steak on the pan and broil for 4 to 6 minutes per side, or until steak is cooked as desired. Let the steak rest for about 5 minutes before carving.

TRIGGER TIP: Chili lime marinade is excellent for chicken or salmon as well.

COOKING TIP: To cook this on the stove, heat 1 tablespoon of butter in a medium saucepan until melted. Cook the steak for 5 to 7 minutes on each side, depending on desired doneness.

PER SERVING: Total Calories: 180; Total Fat: 7g; Saturated Fat: 3g; Cholesterol: 50mg; Sodium: 655mg; Potassium: 45mg; Total Carbohydrate: 2g; Fiber: 0g; Sugars: 1g; Protein: 25g

CINCINNATI-STYLE CHILI

SERVES 8   **PREP TIME** 5 MINUTES   **COOK TIME** 30 MINUTES

Cincinnati-style chili is basically a base of spaghetti combined with ground beef, tomato paste, spices, and cheese. This protein-rich dish is more like gravy than traditional chili. Cincinnati chili has its own lingo. A "two-way" is chili and spaghetti, and a "three-way" is chili, spaghetti, and shredded cheese. A "four-way" is chili, spaghetti, and cheese with *either* beans or chopped onions, and a "five-way" will have beans *and* onions—and will contain more fiber. Speaking of fiber, be sure to serve this chili over whole-wheat spaghetti.

✓ **30-MINUTE**

1 pound lean ground beef (90% lean or higher)

6 cups water

1 (6-ounce) can tomato paste

¼ cup chili powder

1½ tablespoons cocoa powder

1 teaspoon ground cinnamon

1 teaspoon garlic powder

1 teaspoon ground cumin

1 teaspoon allspice

¾ teaspoon salt

¼ teaspoon ground cloves

¼ teaspoon crushed red pepper flakes

⅛ teaspoon freshly ground black pepper

2 tablespoons apple cider vinegar

1 pound whole-wheat spaghetti

1 (16-ounce) bag shredded Cheddar cheese

1. In a large pot over medium-high heat, combine the ground beef, water, and tomato paste.

2. Bring the meat mixture to a boil and cook for 5 minutes, stirring to break up the beef and dissolve the tomato paste.

3. Add the chili powder, cocoa powder, cinnamon, garlic powder, cumin, allspice, salt, cloves, red pepper flakes, black pepper, and vinegar. Reduce the heat to low and cook for 30 minutes.

4. While the chili is cooking, boil water in a large pot. Add the spaghetti noodles and cook for 8 to 10 minutes, or until al dente. Drain the spaghetti and serve ½ to 1 cup of chili over each serving of noodles. Top with 2 tablespoons of shredded cheese per serving.

SUBSTITUTION TIP: You can use ground turkey in place of the beef.

PER SERVING: Total Calories: 560; Total Fat: 25g; Saturated Fat: 14g; Cholesterol: 92mg; Sodium: 669mg; Potassium: 515mg; Total Carbohydrate: 51g; Fiber: 5g; Sugars: 5g; Protein: 35g

PORK STIR-FRY WITH BROWN RICE

SERVES 4   **PREP TIME** 10 MINUTES   **COOK TIME** 20 MINUTES

This colorful dish is a good source of vitamin C and protein, two nutrients that keep your immune system humming. It's simple enough to make for a weeknight meal and nice enough to impress company. Using brown rice instead of white boosts the fiber content of this meal and makes it more filling.

✓ **30-MINUTE**
✓ **GLUTEN-FREE**
✓ **ONE POT**

2 cups water

1 cup brown rice

1 tablespoon corn oil, divided

1 red bell pepper, cut into strips

1 yellow bell pepper, cut into strips

3 green onions, cut into 2-inch pieces

1-pound pork tenderloin, fat trimmed and cut into 1-inch pieces

½ teaspoon salt

½ teaspoon freshly ground black pepper

2 garlic cloves, minced

1 teaspoon ginger paste

¼ cup low-sodium soy sauce

1½ tablespoons brown sugar

1½ tablespoons cornstarch

Brown rice, for serving

Sesame seeds, for topping (optional)

1. Place the water and brown rice in a medium pot and bring to a boil. Cook for 5 minutes, and then turn down heat and simmer for 25 minutes, or until the water is absorbed and the rice is fully cooked. Set aside.

2. Heat 1 teaspoon of the oil in a large skillet over medium heat. Add the red and yellow bell peppers and cook for 3 minutes, or until soft. Add the green onions and cook for 2 minutes. Remove the peppers and onions to a bowl and set aside.

3. In another bowl, season the pork with salt and pepper.

4. Add the remaining 2 teaspoons of oil to the skillet along with the pork. Cook for 5 minutes, or until pork is lightly browned. Add the garlic and ginger and cook for 1 minute. Add the peppers and onions back to the pan.

5. In a small bowl, whisk together the soy sauce, brown sugar, and cornstarch. Pour the sauce over the pork mixture and simmer for 2 to 3 minutes, or until sauce has thickened and top with sesame seeds, if desired. Serve over brown rice.

VARIATION TIP: Use zucchini or chopped broccoli instead of peppers to add more texture, color, and nutrition to the stir-fry.

PER SERVING: Total Calories: 383; Total Fat: 9g; Saturated Fat: 2g; Cholesterol: 65mg; Sodium: 1042mg; Potassium: 333mg; Total Carbohydrate: 51g; Fiber: 3g; Sugars: 6g; Protein: 26g

BEEF TENDERLOIN IN COFFEE MARINADE

SERVES 4 **PREP TIME** 5 MINUTES, PLUS 60 MINUTES TO MARINATE **COOK TIME** 15 MINUTES

Don't toss the leftover coffee from breakfast! Upcycle it into a delicious marinade at dinnertime. Did you know coffee helps prevent gout flare-ups? Coffee has been shown to help lower uric acid levels and is naturally high in antioxidants.

✓ **DIABETIC FRIENDLY**

✓ **GLUTEN-FREE**

✓ **ONE POT**

1 cup black coffee, room temperature

¼ cup balsamic vinegar

¼ cup Dijon mustard

¼ cup packed brown sugar

2 tablespoons olive oil

2 teaspoons freshly ground pepper, divided

1 small onion, chopped

2 garlic cloves, minced

1½ pounds beef tenderloin or skirt steak, fat trimmed, cut into 4 pieces

1 teaspoon salt

1. In a medium bowl, whisk together the coffee, vinegar, mustard, brown sugar, oil, and 1 teaspoon of pepper. Stir in the onion and garlic. Pour half of the marinade into a large resealable plastic bag. Add the steak, seal the bag, and massage to coat. Let the steak sit at room temperature for 1 hour. Cover the rest of the marinade and set aside.

2. Preheat the grill to medium-high heat. Remove steak from the marinade and discard the used marinade. Season steak with salt and the remaining 1 teaspoon of pepper and grill, turning and basting often with reserved marinade, 8 to 10 minutes for medium-rare. Let rest for 10 minutes before slicing.

3. If broiling the steak, set oven rack 5 inches below the broiler element. Place the marinated steak in a broiling pan and broil for 5 to 7 minutes per side, depending on desired doneness.

COOKING TIP: The steak can be marinated a day ahead. Chill, turning occasionally. Keep the reserved marinade chilled. Prior to cooking, bring the steak to room temperature.

PER SERVING: Total Calories: 316; Total Fat: 14g; Saturated Fat: 5g; Cholesterol: 114mg; Sodium: 858mg; Potassium: 701mg; Total Carbohydrate: 4g; Fiber: 1g; Sugars: 1g; Protein: 39g

HONEY GLAZED PORK CHOPS WITH CINNAMON SPICE

SERVES 4 **PREP TIME** 5 MINUTES **COOK TIME** 15 MINUTES

If you're a cinnamon and honey fan, you'll love this quick recipe. Lean pork is a gout-friendly protein source that's high in B vitamins and iron. It can be paired with mashed sweet potatoes and roasted broccoli for a colorful, delicious meal.

✓ 30-MINUTE
✓ DIABETIC FRIENDLY
✓ GLUTEN-FREE
✓ KIDNEY FRIENDLY
✓ ONE POT

¼ cup honey

2 tablespoons yellow mustard

½ teaspoon ground cinnamon

½ teaspoon allspice

Nonstick cooking spray

4 (4-ounce) boneless center-cut pork chops (about ½-inch thick)

½ teaspoon kosher salt

¼ teaspoon freshly ground black pepper

1. In a small bowl, combine the honey, mustard, cinnamon, and allspice.

2. Heat a large nonstick skillet over medium heat and coat it with nonstick cooking spray.

3. Season the pork chops with salt and pepper; then cook for 2 minutes on each side, or until the pork is browned.

4. Reduce the heat to medium, and then add the honey mixture. Cook for 5 minutes, and then turn pork chops and cook another 5 minutes, or until done.

SUBSTITUTION TIP: Ground ginger can be used in place of the allspice.

PER SERVING: Total Calories: 142; Total Fat: 3g; Saturated Fat: 1g; Cholesterol: 50mg; Sodium: 290mg; Potassium: 18mg; Total Carbohydrate: 12g; Fiber: 0g; Sugars: 12g; Protein: 17g

PORK CARNITAS

SERVES 8   **PREP TIME** 5 MINUTES   **COOK TIME** 6 TO 10 HOURS

Pork carnitas are an excellent one-pot meal that can be cooking while you're at work or away all day at a soccer game. This is a gout-, diabetic-, and kidney-friendly recipe that's an excellent source of protein. Shredded pork can be used in tacos or sandwiches.

✓ **DIABETIC FRIENDLY**
✓ **KIDNEY FRIENDLY**
✓ **ONE POT**

4 pounds pork shoulder

2 teaspoons kosher salt

1½ teaspoons freshly ground black pepper

1 tablespoon olive oil

1 teaspoon dried oregano

1 teaspoon ground cumin

1 onion, diced

1 jalapeño pepper, seeded and chopped

4 garlic cloves, minced

¾ cup orange juice

8 whole-wheat tortillas

1 cucumber, seeded and chopped

1. Rub the pork shoulder with salt and pepper. In a small bowl, mix together the oil, oregano, and cumin, and rub this mixture into the pork.

2. Place the seasoned pork in a slow cooker. Add the onion, jalapeño, and garlic. Pour the orange juice over the pork.

3. Set the slow cooker on low for 10 hours or on high for 6 hours.

4. When the pork is done, shred it using two forks. Spoon a few tablespoons of shredded pork on a whole-wheat tortilla and top with 1 tablespoon of chopped cucumbers.

VARIATION TIP: For a tangier taste, try using lime juice instead of orange juice. Corn tortillas or rice can also be used instead of whole-wheat tortillas to make the recipe gluten-free.

COOKING TIP: Pork shoulder can be cooked in the oven too. Preheat the oven to 350°F. Place the seasoned pork in an oven-safe pan, and then pour the orange juice over the pork. Roast pork for 1 hour per pound until cooked to an internal temperature of 145°F.

PER SERVING: Total Calories: 412; Total Fat: 12g; Saturated Fat: 3g; Cholesterol: 130mg; Sodium: 1314mg; Potassium: 145mg; Total Carbohydrate: 28g; Fiber: 4g; Sugars: 3g; Protein: 47g

GARLIC ROSEMARY ROASTED PORK TENDERLOIN

SERVES 8   **PREP TIME** 15 MINUTES, PLUS 2 HOURS TO MARINATE   **COOK TIME** 50 MINUTES

Did you know that crushing garlic and letting it rest for 10 minutes before cooking releases its anti-inflammatory properties? In addition to health benefits, garlic just makes everything *tastier*. This savory recipe combines loads of garlic and rosemary with heart-healthy olive oil to make a delicious rub. The pork can be cooked in a slow cooker or roasted in the oven.

✓ **DIABETIC FRIENDLY**

✓ **GLUTEN-FREE**

✓ **KIDNEY FRIENDLY**

8 garlic cloves, minced and set aside for 10 minutes

¼ cup plus 2 tablespoons olive oil, divided

2 tablespoons dried rosemary

2 teaspoons sea salt

½ teaspoon freshly ground black pepper

2 pounds pork tenderloin

1. In a large bowl, combine the garlic, ¼ cup of oil, rosemary, salt, and pepper. Add the pork tenderloin to the marinade and rub the pork until coated.

2. Refrigerate for at least 2 hours but not longer than 24 hours. Take the pork out to rest at room temperature for 30 minutes before cooking.

3. Preheat the oven to 400°F.

4. In a large oven-safe skillet or Dutch oven, heat the remaining 2 tablespoons of oil over medium-high heat. Brown the pork on all sides, about 5 minutes, before placing it in the oven to roast.

5. Roast the pork for 40 to 45 minutes, or until the inside is no longer pink. Transfer the pork to a large cutting board and let it rest for 5 minutes before cutting.

COOKING TIP: If using a slow cooker, brown the pork for 5 minutes before placing it in the slow cooker, and set on low for 6 to 8 hours. Slice or shred the pork before serving.

PER SERVING: Total Calories: 154; Total Fat: 8g; Saturated Fat: 2g; Cholesterol: 65mg; Sodium: 300mg; Potassium: 13mg; Total Carbohydrate: 1g; Fiber: 0g; Sugars: 0g; Protein: 20g

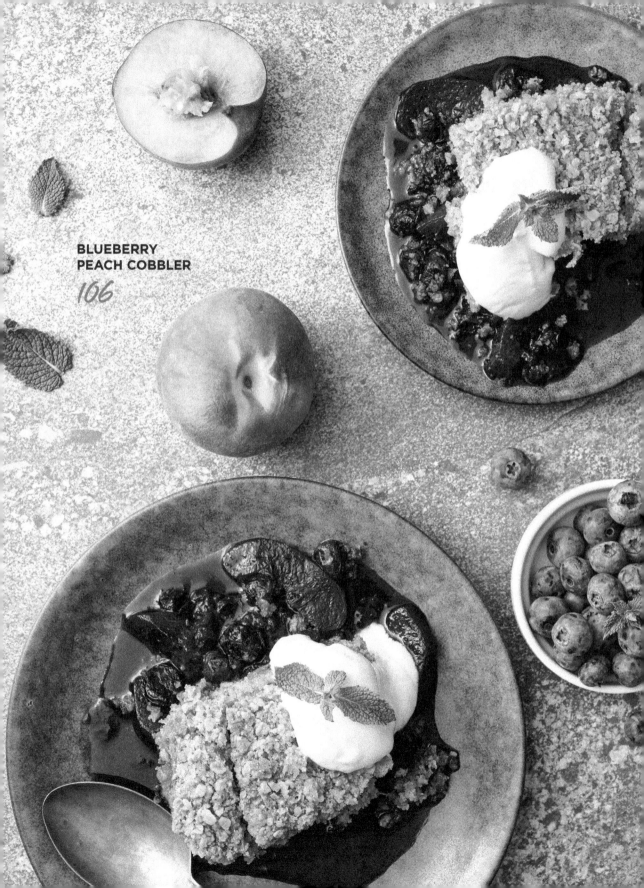

BLUEBERRY PEACH COBBLER

106

8

Desserts

Every good meal deserves a sweet ending. This chapter provides a variety of delicious treats, from fruit-based sweets like Apple Cherry Crumble (page 108) and Baked Pears with Pistachios and Cinnamon (page 107) to decadent ones like Chocolate Raspberry Trifle (page 113) and Tangy Lime Bars with Shortbread Crust (page 114). Every recipe is simple to prepare and even more delightful to eat.

BLUEBERRY PEACH COBBLER

SERVES 8   **PREP TIME** 5 MINUTES   **COOK TIME** 45 MINUTES

You don't have to wait for summer to enjoy this dessert! It's made with frozen blueberries and canned peaches (although you can also use fresh fruit, if you have it). Not only are blueberries and peaches delicious, but they are also very nutritious. Blueberries are high in anti-inflammatory phytochemicals like anthocyanin—which gives the berries their blue hue—and vitamin C. Peaches should also be enjoyed often for their cancer-fighting beta-carotene and vitamin C.

✓ **KIDNEY FRIENDLY**

✓ **VEGETARIAN**

Butter or nonstick cooking spray

2 (15-ounce) cans sliced peaches packed in water, undrained

1 cup frozen blueberries

1 teaspoon lemon zest

¾ cup all-purpose flour

½ cup brown sugar

1 teaspoon baking powder

1 stick salted butter

Whipped cream, for topping (optional)

Fresh mint leaves, for garnish (optional)

1. Preheat the oven to 400°F. Grease or spray a 9-by-9-inch glass baking pan.

2. Place the peaches and their juices into the glass pan.

3. In a small bowl, toss the blueberries with the lemon zest. Pour over the peaches.

4. In a separate bowl, mix the flour, brown sugar, and baking powder. Using a fork or pastry cutter, add the butter to the flour mixture to create a crumble. Cover the fruit mixture evenly with the crumble.

5. Bake for 45 to 60 minutes, or until the fruit is bubbling and the top of the crumble is turning light brown. Cool and allow the filling to thicken. Slice and top with a dollop of whipped cream and garnish with mint leaves, if desired, before serving.

SUBSTITUTION TIP: If you don't have lemon zest, 1 tablespoon of lemon juice can be added to the blueberries for lemony flavor.

PER SERVING: Total Calories: 272; Total Fat: 12g; Saturated Fat: 7g; Cholesterol: 30mg; Sodium: 93mg; Potassium: 106mg; Total Carbohydrate: 41g; Fiber: 2g; Sugars: 30g; Protein: 2g

BAKED PEARS WITH PISTACHIOS AND CINNAMON

SERVES 4   **PREP TIME** 5 MINUTES   **COOK TIME** 15 MINUTES

Take advantage of beautiful pears while they're in season. They've got a sweet, floral taste and grainy texture, not to mention they are a gout-friendly, low-purine fruit. Pears are also a good source of cholesterol-lowering soluble fiber. The pistachios in this dessert add color, taste, and crunch to the pears as well as heart-healthy fat and a small dose of protein. Just like pears, pistachios are low in purines, making them an excellent snack on their own for anyone with gout. I like to serve these pears with vanilla frozen yogurt or butter pecan ice cream for a special treat.

✓ **30-MINUTE**
✓ **GLUTEN-FREE**
✓ **ONE POT**
✓ **VEGAN**

4 pears, quartered

4 teaspoons brown sugar

4½ teaspoons ground cinnamon

¼ cup shelled pistachios, chopped

1. Preheat the oven to 375°F. Line a baking sheet with parchment paper.

2. Place the pears skin-side down on the baking sheet. With a knife, score each pear in a crisscross fashion twice.

3. In a small bowl, mix the brown sugar, cinnamon, and pistachios. Sprinkle ½ teaspoon of the cinnamon-sugar mixture over each pear.

4. Bake for 25 minutes, or until the pears are slightly browned and soft. Serve with vanilla or butter pecan ice cream or frozen yogurt.

SUBSTITUTION TIP: No pears on hand? Try this recipe with fresh apples or peaches for a summer treat.

PER SERVING: Total Calories: 177; Total Fat: 4g; Saturated Fat: 0g; Cholesterol: 0mg; Sodium: 43mg; Potassium: 250mg; Total Carbohydrate: 38g; Fiber: 8g; Sugars: 24g; Protein: 2g

APPLE CHERRY CRUMBLE

SERVES 4 **PREP TIME** 5 MINUTES **COOK TIME** 60 MINUTES

As I mentioned in chapter 1, cherries are known for their high antioxidant and anti-inflammatory properties. I've paired apples with cherries in this recipe to give this dessert a tart surprise. This recipe uses whole-wheat flour and rolled oats to provide a heartier streusel texture in addition to a bit more fiber. Serve this crumble solo or topped with vanilla frozen yogurt.

✓ VEGETARIAN

1 cup whole-wheat flour

½ cup packed brown sugar

½ cup rolled oats

¼ cup chopped pecans

½ teaspoon salt

½ teaspoon pumpkin
 pie spice

1½ sticks cold, unsalted
 butter, cut into cubes

2 pounds (4 cups) fresh or
 frozen cherries, pitted

1 Granny Smith apple,
 cored and chopped into
 1-inch pieces

½ cup white sugar

1 teaspoon apple
 cider vinegar

1 teaspoon vanilla extract

1. Preheat the oven to 350°F. In a large bowl, whisk together the flour, brown sugar, oats, pecans, salt, and pumpkin pie spice. Using a fork or pastry cutter, add the butter to the flour mixture to create a crumble. Press the flour mixture into smaller clumps and chill in the refrigerator for 15 minutes.

2. While the crumble cools, combine the cherries, apple, white sugar, vinegar, and vanilla in an oven-safe skillet (such as cast iron). Cook over medium heat, stirring, for 5 to 7 minutes, or until the mixture bubbles.

3. Spread the crumble evenly over the fruit mixture and bake for one hour, or until the top is golden brown and fruit is bubbly. Serve warm.

SUBSTITUTION TIP: Out of apple cider vinegar? No problem. Balsamic vinegar works just fine.

PER SERVING: Total Calories: 805; Total Fat: 42g; Saturated Fat: 23g; Cholesterol: 91mg; Sodium: 305mg; Potassium: 478mg; Total Carbohydrate: 107g; Fiber: 8g; Sugars: 70g; Protein: 8g

DARK CHOCOLATE ORANGE SURPRISE CAKE

SERVES 8 **PREP TIME** 10 MINUTES **COOK TIME** 25 MINUTES

This is one of those sneaky desserts that you won't believe unless you see the ingredients on the counter. Puréed black beans take the place of flour in this nontraditional cake recipe to add fiber and protein. Orange extract is swapped for vanilla and pairs deliciously with dark chocolate. Using cocoa powder to dust the pan enhances the flavor and keeps the dessert gluten-free.

✓ **GLUTEN-FREE**

✓ **KIDNEY FRIENDLY**

✓ **VEGETARIAN**

Cocoa powder, for dusting

1 (15-ounce) can black beans, drained and rinsed

4 eggs

1 bag semisweet chocolate chips

½ cup white sugar

½ teaspoon baking powder

2 teaspoons orange extract

1. Preheat the oven to 350°F. Grease a 9-inch baking pan and dust it with cocoa powder.

2. Add the black beans and eggs to a food processor and process until completely smooth.

3. Melt the chocolate chips in the microwave or using a double boiler on the stovetop.

4. Add the melted chocolate, sugar, baking powder, and orange extract to the food processor and process until the mixture is smooth.

5. Pour the batter into the prepared pan and bake for 25 to 30 minutes, or until done.

SUBSTITUTION TIP: No black beans on hand? Navy or great northern beans or chickpeas can be used instead.

PER SERVING: Total Calories: 324; Total Fat: 12g; Saturated Fat: 7g; Cholesterol: 82mg; Sodium: 32mg; Potassium: 187mg; Total Carbohydrate: 46g; Fiber: 3g; Sugars: 33g; Protein: 8g

BANANA BUNDT CAKE WITH CINNAMON GLAZE

SERVES 8 **PREP TIME** 15 MINUTES **COOK TIME** 45 MINUTES, PLUS 20 MINUTES TO COOL

Love food, but hate food waste? Me too! If you've got a few spotty or brown bananas, this treat is for you. Using light sour cream reduces fat and calories. Moist, flavorful banana cake pairs so nicely with light cinnamon glaze. While this cake looks beautiful in bundt form, a 9-by-13-inch baking pan works just fine.

✓ **VEGETARIAN**

FOR THE CAKE

Nonstick cooking spray

Flour, for dusting

1½ cups canola or corn oil

1¾ cup white sugar

2 eggs

2 teaspoons almond extract

1 cup light sour cream

3 bananas, mashed

3 cups all-purpose flour

2 teaspoons baking soda

¾ teaspoon salt

FOR THE GLAZE

1 cup powdered sugar

2 tablespoons milk

1 teaspoon vanilla extract

½ teaspoon
ground cinnamon

1. Preheat the oven to 350°F. Spray a Bundt pan with nonstick cooking spray, and dust with flour. Set aside.

2. In a large mixing bowl, combine the oil, white sugar, eggs, almond extract, sour cream, and mashed bananas. Beat with a hand mixer at medium speed until all the ingredients are combined.

3. In a separate mixing bowl, whisk together the flour, baking soda, and salt.

4. Gradually add the flour mixture to the banana mixture and mix on low speed until just combined.

5. Pour the batter evenly into the prepared pan. Bake for 45 to 55 minutes, or until a toothpick inserted into the middle comes out clean. Allow the cake to cool for 20 minutes before flipping over onto a wire rack or large plate to cool completely.

6. To make the glaze, combine the powdered sugar, milk, vanilla extract, and cinnamon in a mixing bowl and beat until a glaze forms. Drizzle glaze over the cake and let set for 10 minutes before serving.

VARIATION TIP: If you don't have any bananas on hand, use 1½ cups of chopped apples to make a cinnamon apple cake.

PER SERVING: Total Calories: 876; Total Fat: 49g; Saturated Fat: 10g; Cholesterol: 54mg; Sodium: 566mg; Potassium: 269mg; Total Carbohydrate: 106g; Fiber: 3g; Sugars: 64g; Protein: 8g

MOCHA CHOCOLATE CHIP COOKIES

MAKES 2½ DOZEN COOKIES   **PREP TIME** 10 MINUTES   **COOK TIME** 15 MINUTES

Coffee fans, rejoice! Here is a chocolate chip recipe just for you. This recipe uses 25 percent less butter than traditional cookie recipes, which helps reduce the saturated fat and calorie content. Reducing fat also gives the cookies a crispier texture. Chopped pecans or walnuts can also be added to the dough if you want more texture and taste in your cookies.

✓ **30-MINUTE**

✓ **KIDNEY FRIENDLY**

✓ **ONE POT**

✓ **VEGETARIAN**

1½ sticks unsalted butter

¾ cup brown sugar

¾ cup white sugar

1 tablespoon instant coffee

2 eggs

1 teaspoon vanilla extract

1 teaspoon baking soda

1 teaspoon salt

2¼ cups all-purpose flour

1 (12-ounce) bag mini
  semisweet chocolate chips

1. Preheat the oven to 375°F.

2. Soften the butter in the microwave for 30 to 45 seconds or on the stove over low heat for 2 to 3 minutes.

3. Place the butter, brown sugar, white sugar, and instant coffee into the bowl of a stand mixer, or use a large bowl and a hand mixer. Beat until the butter and sugar are creamed together.

4. Add the eggs, vanilla, baking soda, and salt and beat until blended. Gradually add the flour to the butter mixture. A tablespoon of flour can be added if the dough is too wet. It should be just slightly sticky.

5. Add the chocolate chips to the dough and blend.

6. Line a sheet pan with parchment paper or a silicone baking mat. Roll dough into 1-inch balls and place 12 to 15 at a time on the sheet pan.

7. Bake for 8 to 10 minutes, or until the cookies are golden brown. Cool for 10 to 15 minutes before serving.

VARIATION TIP: Try peppermint extract in place of vanilla for a cool mint mocha cookie!

PER SERVING (1 COOKIE): Total Calories: 151; Total Fat: 7g; Saturated Fat: 5g; Cholesterol: 22mg; Sodium: 147mg; Potassium: 21mg; Total Carbohydrate: 21g; Fiber: 1g; Sugars: 14g; Protein: 1g

PUMPKIN CAKE WITH CREAM CHEESE ICING

MAKES 16 SERVINGS **PREP TIME** 5 MINUTES **COOK TIME** 30 MINUTES

Pumpkin cake makes a great dessert during the holiday season—or anytime you're in the mood for it. Did you know that in addition to being a fall favorite, pumpkin is a heart-healthy source of potassium and beta-carotene? This recipe includes a savory-sweet cream cheese frosting that's a bit lower in calories and fat than traditional icings.

✓ **KIDNEY FRIENDLY**

✓ **VEGETARIAN**

FOR THE CAKE

1⅔ cup white sugar

1 cup canola or
   vegetable oil

1 (15-ounce) can
   pumpkin purée

4 eggs

2 cups all-purpose flour

2 teaspoons baking powder

1 teaspoon
   ground cinnamon

1 teaspoon allspice

1 teaspoon baking soda

1 teaspoon salt

FOR THE FROSTING

8-ounce reduced-fat
   cream cheese

1 stick butter,
   room temperature

1½ cups powdered sugar

1 teaspoon vanilla extract

1. Preheat the oven to 350°F. Grease and flour a 9-by-13-inch baking pan.

2. In a large bowl, whisk together the sugar, oil, and pumpkin. Add the eggs and stir until blended.

3. In a separate large bowl, whisk together the flour, baking powder, cinnamon, allspice, baking soda, and salt. Add the dry ingredients to the wet ingredients and blend until smooth.

4. Pour the batter into the prepared pan and bake for 30 to 35 minutes, or until a toothpick inserted into the center of the cake comes out clean. Allow the cake to cool for 20 to 30 minutes before frosting.

5. Make the frosting by combining the cream cheese, butter, powdered sugar, and vanilla. Beat the ingredients together until smooth using a hand mixer. If the frosting is too thick, mix in a teaspoon of milk at a time. Once the cake is cooled, frost and serve it.

SUBSTITUTION TIP: The frosting can be left off the cake to reduce fat and calories. Dust the cake lightly with powdered sugar instead.

PER SERVING: Total Calories: 414; Total Fat: 24g; Saturated Fat: 7g; Cholesterol: 68mg; Sodium: 356mg; Potassium: 154mg; Total Carbohydrate: 48g; Fiber: 1g; Sugars: 34g; Protein: 5g

CHOCOLATE RASPBERRY TRIFLE

MAKES 8 SERVINGS   **PREP TIME** 15 MINUTES, PLUS 4 HOURS TO CHILL

There is something decadent about the combination of chocolate and raspberry, and everyone should have a chance to enjoy it at some point or another. This seemingly indulgent dessert is simple to make, fairly low-fat, and includes antioxidant-rich raspberries to boot. This recipe saves time by using a store-bought cake, but cookies or brownies that are a day or two old can also be used up in this dessert. If they are in season, you can use fresh raspberries instead of frozen.

✓ **30-MINUTE**

✓ **VEGETARIAN**

1 (5-ounce) package instant chocolate pudding mix

3 cups 1% or 2% milk, chilled

1 (9-inch) angel food cake, cut into 1-inch pieces

1 (16-ounce) frozen raspberries, thawed

1 container frozen whipped topping, thawed

1. In a medium bowl, place the pudding mix and cold milk and whisk until it thickens.

2. In a glass serving dish or trifle bowl, layer half of the cake pieces, half of the pudding, half of the raspberries, and half of the whipped topping. Repeat the layering process a second time.

3. Cover the bowl and refrigerate for at least 4 hours before serving.

VARIATION TIP: If you have extra Tangy Lime Bars with Shortbread Crust (see page 114) on hand, they make an excellent replacement for the angel food cake with vanilla pudding instead of chocolate. Lime and raspberry are delicious together!

PER SERVING: Total Calories: 300; Total Fat: 4g; Saturated Fat: 2g; Cholesterol: 15mg; Sodium: 421mg; Potassium: 278mg; Total Carbohydrate: 62g; Fiber: 4g; Sugars: 27g; Protein: 7g

TANGY LIME BARS WITH SHORTBREAD CRUST

MAKES 36 SERVINGS   **PREP TIME** 15 MINUTES   **COOK TIME** 40 MINUTES

This classic, refreshing dessert features a tart lime filling in a buttery crust. Lime bars can be served at a church barbecue or your favorite holiday gathering. Fresh or bottled lime juice can be used to make the filling, but lime zest provides most of the flavor.

✓ **KIDNEY FRIENDLY**

✓ **VEGETARIAN**

1 cup salted butter, softened

2 cups white sugar, divided

2¼ cups all-purpose flour, divided

4 eggs

2 limes, juiced

1 teaspoon lime zest

Powdered sugar, for dusting

1. Preheat the oven to 350°F.

2. In a medium bowl, combine the butter, ½ cup of white sugar, and 2 cups of flour. Press this mixture into the bottom of a 9-by-12-inch pan. Bake for 15 to 20 minutes, or until golden brown.

3. While the crust is baking, make the filling. In another bowl, whisk together the remaining 1½ cups of sugar and ¼ cup of flour with the eggs, lime juice, and lime zest. Pour over the baked crust and bake for another 20 minutes, or until done. Allow the bars to cool before cutting.

4. Dust the bars with powdered sugar, and then cut into 2-inch squares.

VARIATION TIP: Serve the lime bars with freshly chopped raspberries on top.

PER SERVING: Total Calories: 130; Total Fat: 6g; Saturated Fat: 3g; Cholesterol: 32mg; Sodium: 43mg; Potassium: 20mg; Total Carbohydrate: 19g; Fiber: 0g; Sugars: 13g; Protein: 2g

PEANUT BUTTER BLONDIES WITH CHOCOLATE DRIZZLE

MAKES 16 SERVINGS   **PREP TIME** 5 MINUTES   **COOK TIME** 20 MINUTES

Savory peanut butter with semisweet chocolate is one of life's greatest pleasures. This recipe has just seven ingredients and can be ready in less than 30 minutes. Serve these blondie bars with a scoop of vanilla or chocolate ice cream for a special treat.

✓ **30-MINUTE**
✓ **DIABETIC FRIENDLY**
✓ **KIDNEY FRIENDLY**
✓ **VEGETARIAN**

½ cup unsalted
  butter, melted

¾ cup brown sugar

1 egg

1 teaspoon vanilla extract

½ cup crunchy
  peanut butter

1 cup all-purpose flour

1 cup mini semisweet
  chocolate chips

1. Preheat the oven to 350°F. Line an 8-by-8-inch baking pan with parchment paper and set aside.

2. In a large bowl, combine the melted butter and brown sugar. Add the egg and vanilla and mix well. Stir in the peanut butter and mix together until completely combined.

3. Stir in the flour. Spread the batter evenly into the prepared baking pan.

4. Bake the brownies for 20 to 25 minutes, or until a toothpick inserted in the center comes out clean. Allow to cool for 20 minutes.

5. While brownies are cooling, melt the chocolate chips in a microwave-safe bowl. Drizzle melted chocolate over the cooled blondies. Chill in the refrigerator to allow the chocolate to harden before cutting and serving.

VARIATION TIP: Try cinnamon in place of vanilla extract for a delicious twist.

PER SERVING: Total Calories: 227; Total Fat: 14g; Saturated Fat: 7g;
Cholesterol: 25mg; Sodium: 84mg; Potassium: 75mg;
Total Carbohydrate: 24g; Fiber: 2g; Sugars: 15g; Protein: 3g

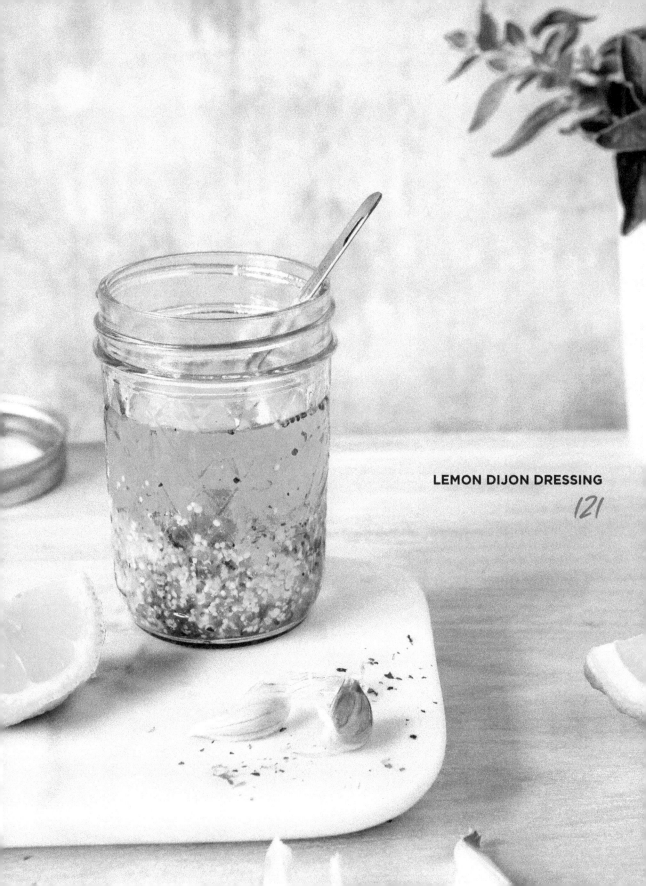

LEMON DIJON DRESSING
121

9

Kitchen Staples, Condiments, and Dressings

Kitchen staples include your go-to salad dressings, marinades, and any sauces that spice up ordinary meats and greens. You'll find deliciously different recipes such as Cumin Lime Salad Dressing (page 118), Simple Marsala Sauce (page 122), and Maple Sriracha Marinade (page 125). Each recipe uses gout-friendly ingredients and has substitutions for alcohol and other ingredients as needed.

CUMIN LIME SALAD DRESSING

SERVES 8   **PREP TIME** 5 MINUTES

Cumin should be in everyone's pantry. This warm, versatile spice is excellent in Indian cuisine as well as Latin American and Middle Eastern dishes. It is a must-have in chili. It is paired with lime juice, a good source of vitamin C, in this unique dressing that can be used as a marinade as well.

✓ **30-MINUTE**
✓ **DIABETIC FRIENDLY**
✓ **GLUTEN-FREE**
✓ **KIDNEY FRIENDLY**
✓ **ONE POT**
✓ **VEGAN**

¼ cup lime juice (fresh or bottled)

¼ cup olive oil

1 teaspoon ground cumin

¼ teaspoon salt

In a small bowl, whisk together the lime juice, oil, cumin, and salt. Dressing can be stored in the refrigerator for up to 1 week.

VARIATION TIP: Lemon juice can be used in place of lime juice. Salt can be omitted if you are on a low-sodium diet.

PER SERVING: Total Calories: 58; Total Fat: 6g; Saturated Fat: 1g; Cholesterol: 0mg; Sodium: 74mg; Potassium: 17mg; Total Carbohydrate: 1g; Fiber: 0g; Sugars: 0g; Protein: 0g

CLASSIC BALSAMIC VINAIGRETTE

SERVES 4 **PREP TIME** 5 MINUTES

If you're trying to reduce your sodium intake, changing your salad dressing is a great place to start. Most commercial dressings contain at least 250mg of sodium per serving. This simple dressing takes minimal time to prepare but can be used on salads or as a marinade for fish, chicken, or steak.

✓ **30-MINUTE**

✓ **DIABETIC FRIENDLY**

✓ **GLUTEN-FREE**

✓ **KIDNEY FRIENDLY**

✓ **ONE POT**

✓ **VEGAN**

2 tablespoons olive or canola oil

2 tablespoons balsamic vinegar

1 tablespoon Dijon mustard

¼ teaspoon salt

In a small bowl, whisk together the oil, vinegar, mustard, and salt. Dressing can be stored in the refrigerator for up to 1 week.

SUBSTITUTION TIP: Corn or vegetable oil can be used in place of canola or olive oil.

PER SERVING: Total Calories: 64; Total Fat: 7g; Saturated Fat: 2g; Cholesterol: 0mg; Sodium: 192mg; Potassium: 11mg; Total Carbohydrate: 0g; Fiber: 0g; Sugars: 0g; Protein: 0g

GINGER SOY MARINADE

SERVES 6 **PREP TIME** 5 MINUTES

You can spend time grating fresh ginger or you can rest your hands and make life simpler by trying ginger paste for this yummy marinade. Ginger makes a delicious combination with garlic and soy sauce and is known to help with digestion. This marinade can be used for fish, pork, chicken, or vegetables.

✓ **30-MINUTE**
✓ **DIABETIC FRIENDLY**
✓ **GLUTEN-FREE**
✓ **ONE POT**
✓ **VEGAN**

3 tablespoons canola oil

3 tablespoons rice wine vinegar or white vinegar

1 teaspoon sesame oil

1 tablespoon low-sodium soy sauce

1 tablespoon ginger paste

1 garlic clove, minced

In a small bowl, whisk together the canola oil, vinegar, sesame oil, soy sauce, ginger, and garlic. Combine with the protein or vegetables of your choice in a large resealable plastic bag and marinate in the refrigerator for at least 30 minutes but not more than 24 hours.

SUBSTITUTION TIP: You can use peanut oil instead of sesame oil. They'll taste similar when cooking.

VARIATION TIP: Want to turn up the heat in this marinade? Add ¼ teaspoon of red pepper flakes or cayenne pepper.

PER SERVING: Total Calories: 79; Total Fat: 8g; Saturated Fat: 1g; Cholesterol: 0mg; Sodium: 100mg; Potassium: 20mg; Total Carbohydrate: 1g; Fiber: 0g; Sugars: 0g; Protein: 0g

LEMON DIJON DRESSING

SERVES 8   **PREP TIME** 8 MINUTES

Dijon mustard is underrated! When making a dressing using mustard, it's best to whisk it *first* before adding the other ingredients as this will help emulsify (blend) the dressing better. Lemon juice, honey, and tarragon provide a fresh flavor to any salad or vegetable.

✓ **30-MINUTE**

✓ **DIABETIC FRIENDLY**

✓ **GLUTEN-FREE**

✓ **KIDNEY FRIENDLY**

✓ **ONE POT**

✓ **VEGAN**

1½ tablespoons
Dijon mustard

¼ cup fresh or bottled
lemon juice

1 teaspoon apple
cider vinegar

2 teaspoons honey

¾ cup canola oil

2 garlic cloves, minced

1 teaspoon dried tarragon

½ teaspoon salt

½ teaspoon freshly ground
black pepper

In a small bowl, whisk the mustard briefly to loosen. Whisk in the lemon juice, vinegar, honey, oil, garlic, tarragon, salt, and pepper. Dressing can be stored in the refrigerator for up to 1 week.

VARIATION TIP: Dried oregano or basil can be used in place of tarragon to modify the flavor.

PER SERVING: Total Calories: 192; Total Fat: 21g; Saturated Fat: 2g; Cholesterol: 0mg; Sodium: 185mg; Potassium: 22mg; Total Carbohydrate: 2g; Fiber: 0g; Sugars: 1g; Protein: 0g

SIMPLE MARSALA SAUCE

SERVES 4   **PREP TIME** 5 MINUTES   **COOK TIME** 15 MINUTES

Marsala sauce gets its name from the marsala wine used in the recipe, but you can easily swap out the wine for chicken or vegetable broth if you'd like to make it alcohol-free. What gives this sauce texture, fiber, and flavor are the other ingredients, including garlic, shallots, and fresh mushrooms. This tasty sauce can be used over chicken, pasta, or pork.

✓ **30-MINUTE**

✓ **DIABETIC FRIENDLY**

✓ **ONE POT**

3 tablespoons olive oil

2 shallots, diced

½ pound fresh button mushrooms, sliced

3 garlic cloves, minced

2 tablespoons flour

½ cup marsala wine

1½ cups low-sodium beef broth

1. Heat the oil in a medium saucepan. Add the shallots, mushrooms, and garlic, and sauté until mushrooms are soft and shallots are translucent, about 5 minutes.

2. Whisk in the flour and cook for 1 minute. Add the wine to the saucepan and whisk until thoroughly combined. Add the beef broth to the pan and simmer on low heat for 5 to 7 minutes, or until the sauce thickens.

SUBSTITUTION TIP: A small white or yellow onion can be used if you don't have shallots.

PER SERVING: Total Calories: 154; Total Fat: 11g; Saturated Fat: 2g; Cholesterol: 0mg; Sodium: 174mg; Potassium: 248mg; Total Carbohydrate: 7g; Fiber: 1g; Sugars: 1g; Protein: 4g

CHILI GARLIC PEANUT SAUCE

SERVES 4   **PREP TIME** 5 MINUTES   **COOK TIME** 10 MINUTES

If you think peanut butter is only good on toast or for kid's lunches, you are missing out! Peanut butter makes a seriously tasty sauce that can be used on noodles, chicken skewers, spring rolls, and more. It's also a vegan source of protein and heart-healthy monounsaturated fat. This easy recipe combines peanut butter with tangy lime juice, spicy chili garlic paste, and savory soy sauce. You'll want to use it over and over again.

✓ **30-MINUTE**

✓ **DIABETIC FRIENDLY**

✓ **ONE POT**

✓ **VEGAN**

½ cup peanut butter (smooth or crunchy)

2 tablespoons low-sodium soy sauce

2 tablespoons lime juice

1 to 2 teaspoons chili garlic paste

¼ cup water, to thin

In a medium saucepan over low heat, whisk together all the ingredients. Simmer for 5 to 10 minutes, or until the sauce is well blended. If the sauce seems too thick, add the water, a tablespoon at a time, until desired consistency is reached.

SUBSTITUTION TIP: If you need a nut-free sauce, you can use sunflower butter instead.

VARIATION TIP: Add 1 to 2 teaspoons of honey to the sauce to make it sweeter.

PER SERVING: Total Calories: 195; Total Fat: 16g; Saturated Fat: 3g; Cholesterol: 0mg; Sodium: 588mg; Potassium: 222mg; Total Carbohydrate: 8g; Fiber: 2g; Sugars: 4g; Protein: 9g

LEMON BUTTER HERB SAUCE

SERVES 4   **PREP TIME** 5 MINUTES   **COOK TIME** 10 MINUTES

Sauces need not take your whole day to prepare to look and taste fancy. You can make this sauce anytime for fish, chicken, steak, pasta, or potatoes. Chopped fresh parsley adds a finishing touch to the sauce, but fresh dill or dried tarragon or rosemary could be used too.

✓ **30-MINUTE**
✓ **DIABETIC FRIENDLY**
✓ **GLUTEN-FREE**
✓ **KIDNEY FRIENDLY**
✓ **ONE POT**

1 tablespoon olive oil

4 garlic cloves, minced

¼ cup lemon juice

2 tablespoons white wine

2 tablespoons butter

2 tablespoons fresh
  parsley, chopped

Heat the oil in a medium saucepan and add the garlic. Sauté for 1 minute, or until the garlic is lightly browned. Add the lemon juice, white wine, and butter and cook until the butter is melted. Pour the sauce into a small mixing bowl and mix in the fresh parsley.

SUBSTITUTION TIP: Leave out the wine and use chicken broth instead to make an alcohol-free sauce.

PER SERVING: Total Calories: 96; Total Fat: 9g; Saturated Fat: 4g; Cholesterol: 15mg; Sodium: 46mg; Potassium: 50mg; Total Carbohydrate: 2g; Fiber: 0g; Sugars: 0g; Protein: 0g

MAPLE SRIRACHA MARINADE

SERVES 4   **PREP TIME** 5 MINUTES

Sriracha sauce is known for its combination of chili peppers, garlic, vinegar, and other spices. Pairing spicy sriracha with sweet maple syrup makes a tangy marinade for pork, chicken, meatballs, or vegetables.

✓ **30-MINUTE**
✓ **DIABETIC FRIENDLY**
✓ **ONE POT**
✓ **VEGAN**
✓ **VERY HIGH SODIUM**

¼ cup sriracha sauce

¼ cup pure maple syrup

2 tablespoons low-sodium soy sauce

1 tablespoon honey

½ cup chopped cilantro

In a medium bowl, combine the sriracha, maple syrup, soy sauce, and honey. Stir in the chopped cilantro to the sriracha sauce. Combine with the protein or vegetables of your choice in a large resealable plastic bag and marinate in the refrigerator for at least 30 minutes but not more than 24 hours.

VARIATION TIP: This sauce can be used for meatballs as an appetizer. Prepare the sauce as noted but leave out the cilantro. Place the sauce in a slow cooker. Add 20 to 25 frozen meatballs and cook on low for 6 to 8 hours.

PER SERVING: Total Calories: 72; Total Fat: 0g; Saturated Fat: 0g; Cholesterol: 0mg; Sodium: 823mg; Potassium: 74mg; Total Carbohydrate: 18g; Fiber: 0g; Sugars: 17g; Protein: 1g

Purine Level Chart

The following table is meant to help you choose foods lower in purines to prevent a gout attack. Ideally, your intake of purines should be below 710mg per day.

FOOD	PURINE CONTENT (IN MG) PER 100 GRAMS (3.5 OUNCES) FOOD
PEPPERS, RED	6.0
POTATO	6.0
CHEESE, CHEDDAR	6.4
PLAIN YOGURT	7.0
CUCUMBERS	7.3
CHERRIES	7.5
BLUEBERRIES	8.0
PEACH	8.0
COTTAGE CHEESE	9.4
RICE, WHITE	10.0
BANANA	11.0
TOMATO	11.0
PEAR	12.0
AVOCADO	13.0
LETTUCE, ICEBERG	13.0
APPLE	14.0
BREAD, WHEAT OR WHITE	14.0
RICE, BROWN	15.0

CARROTS	17.0
GREEN BEANS	18.0
RASPBERRIES	18.0
KIWI	19.0
ORANGE	19.0
PINEAPPLE	19.0
STRAWBERRIES	21.0
ASPARAGUS	23.0
SUMMER SQUASH	24.0
WALNUTS	25.0
GRAPES	27.0
CANTALOUPE	33.0
BREAD, WHOLE-GRAIN	35.0
CABBAGE, SAVOY	37.0
PASTA	40.0
OATMEAL	42.0
KALE	48.0
CAULIFLOWER	51.0
SWEET CORN	52.0
BEEF, LEAN	58.0
SPINACH	57.0
SHRIMP	61.0
PEAS, GREEN	62.0
COD	63.0
PORK TENDERLOIN	63.0
PRUNES	64.0

SALMON	68.0
BRUSSELS SPROUTS	69.0
APRICOT	73.0
BEANS, WHITE	75.0
BROCCOLI	81.0
HAM	83.0
PORK SHOULDER ROAST	83.0
TROUT	87.0
HOT DOGS	89.0
TUNA	107.0
BEEF, FILLET	110.0
BEEF, SHOULDER	110.0
BEEF, CHUCK	120.0
CHICKEN LEG WITH SKIN	125.0
SCALLOPS	136.0
HADDOCK	139.0
VEAL FILLET	140.0
SUNFLOWER SEEDS	143.0
PORK CHOP WITH BONE	145.0
TURKEY WITH SKIN	150.0
MUSSELS	154.0
CHICKEN BREAST WITH SKIN	175.0
TUNA IN OIL	290.0
SARDINES IN OIL	480.0

List adapted from https://elevatehealthaz.com/wp-content/Purine%20Table.pdf

Measurement Conversions

	US STANDARD	US STANDARD (OUNCES)	METRIC (APPROXIMATE)
VOLUME EQUIVALENTS (LIQUID)	2 TABLESPOONS	1 FL. OZ.	30 ML
	¼ CUP	2 FL. OZ.	60 ML
	½ CUP	4 FL. OZ.	120 ML
	1 CUP	8 FL. OZ.	240 ML
	1½ CUPS	12 FL. OZ.	355 ML
	2 CUPS OR 1 PINT	16 FL. OZ.	475 ML
	4 CUPS OR 1 QUART	32 FL. OZ.	1 L
	1 GALLON	128 FL. OZ.	4 L
VOLUME EQUIVALENTS (DRY)	⅛ TEASPOON		0.5 ML
	¼ TEASPOON		1 ML
	½ TEASPOON		2 ML
	¾ TEASPOON		4 ML
	1 TEASPOON		5 ML
	1 TABLESPOON		15 ML
	¼ CUP		59 ML
	⅓ CUP		79 ML
	½ CUP		118 ML
	⅔ CUP		156 ML
	¾ CUP		177 ML
	1 CUP		235 ML
	2 CUPS OR 1 PINT		475 ML
	3 CUPS		700 ML
	4 CUPS OR 1 QUART		1 L
	½ GALLON		2 L
	1 GALLON		4 L
WEIGHT EQUIVALENTS	½ OUNCE		15 G
	1 OUNCE		30 G
	2 OUNCES		60 G
	4 OUNCES		115 G
	8 OUNCES		225 G
	12 OUNCES		340 G
	16 OUNCES OR 1 POUND		455 G

	FAHRENHEIT (F)	CELSIUS (C) (APPROXIMATE)
OVEN TEMPERATURES	250°F	120°C
	300°F	150°C
	325°F	180°C
	375°F	190°C
	400°F	200°C
	425°F	220°C
	450°F	230°C

Resources

Here are some great resources for you to learn more about diet, gout, and general health:

American College of Rheumatology is a professional membership organization committed to improving the care of patients with rheumatic disease. Founded in 1934, this nonprofit organization serves more than 8,400 physicians, health professionals, and scientists. The ACR supports its members by providing education and research.

https://www.rheumatology.org/I-Am-A/Patient-Caregiver/Diseases-Conditions/Gout

American Kidney Fund provides information on the correlation between kidney disease and gout. Included is a quiz to test your knowledge of gout.

https://www.kidneyfund.org

Drugs.com provides an overview of gout and treatment options, including recommended medications to consider.

https://www.drugs.com/slideshow/gout-1159

Elevate Health is the website of Dr. L. Markham McHenry, a doctor of osteopathy. Included is this comprehensive list of low-, medium-, and high-purine foods to help you better plan meals.

https://elevatehealthaz.com/wp-content/Purine%20Table.pdf

Gout Education Society is a nonprofit organization of health care professionals aiming to help those with gout learn about their condition. The site provides a patient-centered quiz that will tailor information based on your answers.

https://gouteducation.org

Harvard Health Publishing, from Harvard Medical School, provides an article outlining causes, predisposing factors, symptoms, complications, treatment, and prevention.

https://www.health.harvard.edu/newsletter_article/all-about-gout

National Institute of Arthritis and Musculoskeletal and Skin Diseases, an organization supporting research into the causes, treatment, and prevention of arthritis and musculoskeletal and skin diseases, provides detailed information on gout: what it is, who typically gets it, symptoms, causes, tests, and treatments.

https://www.niams.nih.gov/health-topics/gout

U.S. Department of Agriculture (USDA) provides tips and ideas to help people build a food plan to meet their individual goals.

www.choosemyplate.gov

References

American Heart Association. "Fish and Omega-3 Fatty Acids." Accessed December 1, 2019. https://www.heart.org/en/healthy-living/healthy-eating /eat-smart/fats/fish-and-omega-3-fatty-acids.

Arthritis Foundation. "What Is Gout?" Accessed December 1, 2019. https://www .arthritis.org/about-arthritis/types/gout/what-is-gout.php.

Caliceti, C., et al. "Fructose Intake, Serum Uric Acid, and Cardiometabolic Disorders: A Critical Review." *Nutrients* 9, no. 4 (2017): 395. doi:10.3390 /nu9040395.

Khanna, Dinesh, et al. "American College of Rheumatology Guidelines for Management of Gout. Part 1: Systematic Nonpharmacologic and Pharmacologic Therapeutic Approaches to Hyperuricemia." *Arthritis Care and Research* 64, no. 10 (2012): 1431–46. doi:10.1002/acr.21772.

Konshin, Victor. *Beating Gout: A Sufferer's Guide to Living Pain Free.* Williamsville, NY: Ayerware Publishing, 2009.

National Heart, Lung, and Blood Institute. "DASH Eating Plan." Accessed December 1, 2019. https://www.nhlbi.nih.gov/health-topics/dash-eating-plan.

Index

Acknowledgments

I have quite a few people to acknowledge for this book. For starters, I'd like to acknowledge my family for their support in my writing this cookbook. To my husband and best friend, Ryan Andrews, who cheered me on and kept the coffee flowing while I worked. And to my daughters, Iris and Maria Andrews, who tried countless recipes for "quality assurance purposes," as we like to say in our house. They also kept the house quiet and left me alone while I hid behind my laptop. I'd also like to acknowledge the help, support, and encouragement of my editor, Erum Khan. I cannot say enough good things about her. She always provided me with speedy, positive feedback and the confidence for me to write my first cookbook. I'd like to thank my mom, who fed me well and helped me appreciate good food. And finally, I wish my dad, Frank Cicciarello, were alive to share the news with and thank in person. I am forever grateful for his sense of humor and love of food that he passed on to me. He would have been so proud to see that I'd written a cookbook.

About the Author

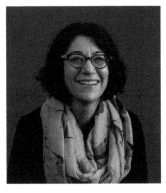

Lisa Cicciarello Andrews is a native of Youngstown, Ohio, and grew up enjoying great Italian food. An interest in people, food, and health led her to become a registered dietitian.

Lisa worked for the VA Medical Center as a clinical dietitian and taught nutrition at the University of Cincinnati for several years. She started Sound Bites Nutrition in 2008 to share her knowledge through counseling, cooking demos, teaching, and freelance writing. Her friends affectionately call her "nutrigirl."

Lisa is the president of the Ohio Academy of Nutrition & Dietetics and served on the Ohio board and Greater Cincinnati Dietetic Association as chair of professional issues and media chair. In 2002, she won the Ohio Recognized Young Dietitian of the Year Award. In 2017, Lisa received the Ohio Recognized Dietitian of the Year Award.

As a person with rheumatoid arthritis, she was an active volunteer for the Arthritis Foundation and was awarded the Arthritis Foundation's Adult Honoree in 2016. Lisa founded People's Pantry Cincy—a program started in 2016 through a philanthropic grant. Being a "word neRD" and passionate about food justice, she designed Lettuce Beet Hunger—food pun swag where a portion of the proceeds support food insecurity programs.

Lisa resides in Cincinnati with her husband, Ryan, daughters, Iris and Maria, and their cat, Snickers. Learn more about her at SoundBitesNutrition.com.

Printed in the USA
CPSIA information can be obtained
at www.ICGtesting.com
LVHW071316261023
762046LV00001B/6